Endodontics

Endodontics
Problem-Solving in Clinical Practice

TR Pitt Ford, BDS, PhD, FDS RCPS
JS Rhodes, BDS, MSc, MRD RCS, MFGDP
HE Pitt Ford, FDS RCS

Department of Conservative Dentistry
Guy's, King's and St Thomas' Dental Institute
King's College London
London, UK

Martin Dunitz

© 2002 Martin Dunitz Ltd, a member of the Taylor & Francis group

First published in the United Kingdom in 2002
by Martin Dunitz Ltd, The Livery House, 7–9 Pratt Street, London NW1 0AE

Tel: +44 (0) 20 74822202
Fax: +44 (0) 20 72670159
E-mail: info@dunitz.co.uk
Website: http://www.dunitz.co.uk

Although every effort has been made to ensure that all owners of copyright material have been acknowledged in this publication, we would be glad to acknowledge in subsequent reprints or editions any omissions brought to our attention.

Although every effort has been made to ensure that drug doses and other information are presented accurately in this publication, the ultimate responsibility rests with the prescribing physician. Neither the publishers nor the authors can be held responsible for errors or for any consequences arising from the use of information contained herein. For detailed prescribing information or instructions on the use of any product or procedure discussed herein, please consult the prescribing information or instructional material issued by the manufacturer.

A CIP record for this book is available from the British Library.

ISBN 1-85317-695-8

Distributed in the United States and Canada by:
Thieme New York
333 Seventh Avenue
New York, NY 10001

Distributed in the rest of the world by:
ITPS Limited
Cheriton House
North Way
Andover, Hampshire SP10 5BE, UK
Tel: +44 (0)1264 332424
E-mail: reception@itps.co.uk

Composition by Wearset Ltd, Boldon, Tyne & Wear

Printed and bound in Singapore by Kyodo Printing Pte Ltd

CONTENTS

Acknowledgements   vi
Preface   vii

1   History, diagnosis and treatment planning   1

2   Three-dimensional root canal anatomy   27

3   Preparation prior to endodontics   45

4   Isolation   65

5   Root canal preparation   79

6   Irrigation and medication   111

7   Obturation techniques   121

8   Root canal retreatment   137

9   Restoration of the endodontically treated tooth   149

10   Complex endodontic problems   165

11   Endodontic care of permanent teeth in children   179

12   Endodontic emergencies   195

Index   201

ACKNOWLEDGEMENTS

The authors wish to thank the following for kind permission to reproduce figures:
Dr M Mohammed (Figures 1.4 and 1.5)
Schick Technologies Inc. (Figure 1.54)
Dr J Lynch (Figure 2.3)
Mr D Pittman (Figure 8.1)
Dr E Sheehy (Figure 11.1).

Figures 1.56, 1.57 and 5.19 are from TR Pitt Ford
Figures 11.4–11.18 are from HE Pitt Ford
All other figures are from JS Rhodes.

John Rhodes would like to acknowledge the contributions made by the following people during the writing of this book:
Neil Conduit of QED, Douglas Pittman of DP Medical, Stuart Clark of Clark Dental, and Kerr UK, who all loaned equipment for photography
The patients and staff at Heath House Dental Health Centre, many of whom agreed to be photographed for illustrative material
John Lynch and Charlie Bird, for their expertise in Micro Computed Tomography
Dr Chris Stock, an endodontic mentor, and my wife, Sarah, who supported me patiently throughout the many hours spent word-processing.

PREFACE

This book has been primarily written for the practising dental practitioner, who would like to be updated in modern clinical endodontics, although it will also be of benefit for practitioners with a special interest in endodontics. With the rise in patient expectations about retaining endodontically involved posterior teeth as well as anteriors, busy dental practitioners need to be aware of current views on diagnosis and treatment.

A problem-solving approach has been adopted since patients present with individual problems, which require predictable and effective solutions. Considerable emphasis is placed on arriving at a reliable diagnosis, and making both the process and the outcome of treatment predictable. With practitioners increasingly presented with patients who have failed root canal treatment, a section is devoted to the effective management of these cases. The days of a 'try it and see' approach have passed; practitioners are now expected to make the correct diagnosis and carry out the appropriate treatment to a high standard, or to refer the patient to a suitably trained person who can.

The book is profusely illustrated to help the reader understand the conditions and techniques being described. The text has been written in an easy-to-read style devoid of original references, but further reading is included at the end of chapters. The authors hope that patients will be the main beneficiaries and that those practitioners who have struggled with root canal treatment will now find their work easier.

TR Pitt Ford
JS Rhodes
HE Pitt Ford

1 HISTORY, DIAGNOSIS AND TREATMENT PLANNING

CONTENTS • Introduction • Surgical Sieve • Medical History • A Medical History Proforma • Infective Endocarditis • Antibiotic Prophylaxis • Patients at Risk of Infective Endocarditis • Chief Complaint • History of Present Complaint • Dental History • Social History • Extraoral Examination • Intraoral Examination • Special Tests • Radiography • Diagnosis • Further Reading

INTRODUCTION

General dental practitioners routinely manage the sequelae of pulpal and periapical inflammation. Differential diagnosis of facial pain can however be very challenging. The patient with endodontic disease will not necessarily present with toothache, and a pain that may at first appear to be of endodontic origin could be referred from elsewhere or even be psychogenic. A careful and methodical approach to history taking, examination and applying special tests will save time and expense at a later date. Cutting corners can unfortunately lead to embarrassing mistakes, and possibly litigation.

Using a surgical sieve to aid history taking and examination is not an original method, but is an invaluable approach for diagnosis in dentistry.

SURGICAL SIEVE

A typical surgical sieve will include the following headings:

- Biographical details
- Medical history
- Chief complaint
- History of present complaint
- Dental history
- Social history
- Extraoral examination
- Intraoral examination
- Special tests
- Radiographs
- Diagnosis
- Treatment plan

MEDICAL HISTORY

There are virtually no medical contraindications to routine endodontic treatment. Debilitating disease, recent myocardial infarction and uncontrolled diabetes will delay treatment. The dental practitioner may require further advice from the patient's medical practitioner on the pharmacology associated with complex drug regimes before embarking on treatment. Fortunately, most patients that present in the dental surgery with systemic disease are well controlled and pose no problem to routine treatment.

A thorough and complete medical history should be taken when the patient has an initial consultation; this is then updated regularly at subsequent appointments. Working from a proforma is one of the most efficient and easiest methods. Vital questions are not overlooked, and it is easy to update at following appointments. Points of interest can be highlighted for all staff treating the patient, and may be particularly useful in an emergency situation.

More frequently patients present with allergies – those to antibiotics and latex are becoming more common. Obviously prescribing patterns should be consistent with any allergy, and it is now possible to use non-latex gloves and rubber dam. The emergency treatment of anaphylaxis is discussed later.

A MEDICAL HISTORY PROFORMA

CONFIDENTIAL – MEDICAL HISTORY

To be completed by patient (delete as appropriate)

FULL NAME ....

DATE OF BIRTH ....../ ....../...... OCCUPATION ....

WHO IS YOUR REGISTERED MEDICAL PRACTITIONER? ....

ADDRESS OF MEDICAL PRACTITIONER..

....

1. Have you ever had Rheumatic Fever?	Yes	No
2. Do you have Heart Trouble or High Blood Pressure?	Yes	No
3. Do you have Chest Trouble?	Yes	No
4. Have you had Jaundice or Hepatitis, or been refused as a blood donor?	Yes	No
5. Have you ever had severe bleeding that needed special treatment after an injury or dental extraction?	Yes	No
6. Is there any family history of Bleeding Disorders?	Yes	No
7. Are you taking any Drugs, Tablets, or Medicines?	Yes	No
If 'Yes' please list		
8. Do you suffer from any Allergies (e.g. Penicillin)?	Yes	No
If 'Yes' please list		
9. Are you Diabetic?	Yes	No
10. Do you have any history of Epilepsy?	Yes	No
11. Have you had any a) Serious Illnesses or Operations?	Yes	No
or b) Adverse reactions to Local or General Anaesthesia?	Yes	No
12. Have you come into contact with anybody who has AIDS or is HIV positive?	Yes	No
13. (Females only) Are you pregnant?	Yes	No

Please add **anything** else you feel might be of importance:

DATE CHECKED

INFECTIVE ENDOCARDITIS

There is general consensus on the recommendations for the prevention of infective endocarditis following dentistry.

A working party of the British Society for Antimicrobial Chemotherapy advocated that the only dental procedures likely to produce a significant bacteraemia were extractions, scaling or surgery involving the gingivae. Significant bacteraemia was unlikely to be produced from root canal instrumentation. There are studies in the endodontic literature that support this. Only gross over-preparation beyond the apex of the tooth and into periapical tissues has produced a bacteraemia. Clinical conditions and presentation vary, and if in doubt a practitioner should contact the patient's general medical practitioner or physician for advice and a second opinion. It may for instance be prudent to provide antibiotic prophylaxis where a tooth is acutely infected or there is significant associated periodontal disease.

ANTIBIOTIC PROPHYLAXIS

Procedures under Local Anaesthetic

Patients who are not allergic to penicillin and have not been prescribed a penicillin more than once in the preceding 4 weeks:

Amoxycillin
Adults: 3g single oral dose 1 hour prior to procedure (this should be supervised, as there is a risk of anaphylaxis)
Children 5–10 years: half adult dose
Children under 5 years: quarter adult dose

A second dose is recommended 6–8 hours later to ensure adequate cover in high-risk patients.

Patients allergic to penicillin or who have had penicillin prescribed within the preceding 4 weeks:

Clindamycin
Adults: 600mg single oral dose 1 hour prior to treatment (this should be supervised)
Children 5–10 years: half the adult dose
Children under 5 years: quarter the adult dose

PATIENTS AT RISK OF INFECTIVE ENDOCARDITIS

- A known history of rheumatic fever
- Congenital heart disease
- Murmurs associated with cardiac disease
- Valve replacements
- Patients who have previously suffered an attack of infective endocarditis (this is more common in diabetics, IV drug abusers and patients on haemodialysis)
- Patients deemed to be at risk by their physician

Patients who have undergone bypass grafting or heart transplant are not considered to be at risk of endocarditis; but it would be wise to seek a medical opinion if in doubt.

The risk of bacteraemia can be reduced quite simply by using a 0.2% chlorhexidine mouthwash preoperatively. The solution should be swilled around the mouth for at least one minute before endodontic treatment or used three times daily, starting 24 hours prior to treatment. Chlorhexidine mouthwash significantly reduces the bacterial load in the oral cavity. The patient will be best served by well-planned and well-executed treatment, as opposed to ineffective root canal treatment. Antibiotic cover is obviously required for at-risk patients undergoing surgical endodontic procedures and replantation of teeth.

CHIEF COMPLAINT

This is the opportunity for the general practitioner to let the patient describe a dental problem as it appears to him/her. You may start with 'Tell me about your problem' or 'How can I help?' Allowing time to listen to the patient in a busy schedule can pay dividends in reaching the correct diagnosis swiftly and avoiding embarrassing mistakes. A distressed patient will be put at ease, and conversation can then lead into more detailed discussion.

HISTORY OF PRESENT COMPLAINT

The discussion is now carefully guided to glean further more detailed and important facts without pre-empting an answer. Leading questions should be avoided.

When did the pain or problem start?

Does anything make the pain better or worse? Application of heat, cloves or pressure may have eased the pain. Have any analgesics been taken? Large doses of anti-inflammatory drugs can depress any discomfort and could alter the practitioner's prescription of further analgesics.

Relieving factors. Lying down, hot water bottles, whisky, and sucking on an aspirin tablet are often used by patients in an attempt to relieve pain!

The frequency of painful episodes. Do pains come and go, or is there a continuous ache? Pain when chewing could be due to apical periodontitis, a cracked cusp or an overbuilt filling.

Intensity. Has the patient been kept awake at night?

Location. An irreversibly pulpitic tooth may not be easily identified by the patient, as the pain can be referred or radiate. Referral of pain occurs along the jaw of the same side, from maxilla to mandible and vice versa, but never across the midline. A tooth with acute apical periodontitis is often tender to bite on and can therefore be identified easily.

Duration. Spontaneous aching and throbbing is often indicative of an irreversible pulpitis or acute apical periodontitis. A tooth is classified as chronic if it is symptomless; this does not however refer to the cell types histologically.

Postural changes. Does the pain increase when lying down or bending over?

Does anything trigger the pain? Pain of short duration following stimulation with hot or cold can often be due to a reversible pulpitis, as with a leaking or recent restoration. Pain lasting several minutes, especially after a hot stimulus, may suggest an irreversible pulpitis.

Quality of pain. Is it sharp, stabbing, radiating, throbbing or dull?

DENTAL HISTORY

Is the patient a regular attender? Will he/she be motivated enough to have the endodontically treated tooth restored, or would extraction be a better course of treatment?

Has he/she presented in pain? If so, how bad is it? Has it kept him/her awake? Ask the patient to grade it on a scale of 1 to 10.

Is the patient particularly nervous of dentistry? Is there a history of difficult extractions or a particularly problematic root canal treatment? Referral to a specialist colleague may be necessary.

Has the patient recently had any restorations placed? Overbuilt or deep fillings may be associated with transient pain after placement.

SOCIAL HISTORY

A social history may be helpful when symptoms and signs do not seem to fit the history of dental pain. The highly distressed, depressed or stressed individual may present with an atypical or psychologically derived pain.

EXTRAORAL EXAMINATION

Palpation

Lymph nodes can be gently palpated with the fingertips. Lymphadenopathy of the submandibular lymph nodes could be an indication of infection in the oral cavity. Tenderness may indicate a site of acute inflammation deep to the skin (Fig. 1.1).

Facial Swelling

Are there any signs of acute inflammation – heat, swelling, redness, pain, loss of function – and does the patient have a raised body temperature?

Does the patient feel that his/her face is swollen in any way? Ask patients to look in a mirror and point to any perceived swelling. The practitioner can assess the facial contour in profile and by looking down the bridge of the nose from above to see any asymmetry in the nasolabial folds (Figs. 1.2, 1.3). Facial

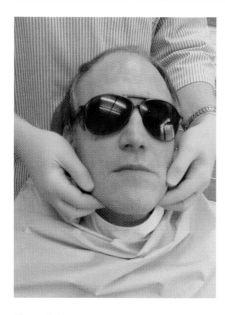

Figure 1.1

Palpation of the submandibular lymph nodes. The clinician is positioned behind the patient and palpates the nodes gently with finger tips.

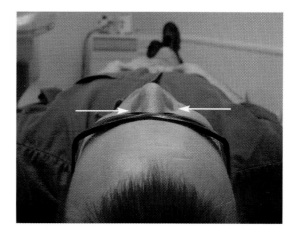

Figure 1.3

Asymmetry in the right nasolabial folds is more visible when viewed from above.

asymmetry can be due to guarding of painful tissues.

External Sinus Tracts

Rarely, a sinus tract leading from an abscess at the apex of a tooth can point externally; this is sometimes seen in the mandibular or maxillary incisor regions (Figs. 1.4, 1.5). The tracts point as a spot on the chin or just inside the nares respectively. The spot does not heal, and may discharge pus.

INTRAORAL EXAMINATION

Ease of access: Is it possible for the patient to open his/her mouth sufficiently wide for root canal treatment? If two fingers can be placed between the maxillary and mandibular incisor tips then it should be possible to instrument most teeth (Fig. 1.6).

General condition of the mouth: Is the mouth in good health or neglected? Are there heavy plaque deposits and evidence of gross periodontal disease (Fig. 1.7)? Are restorations of good quality, or are the margins overhanging

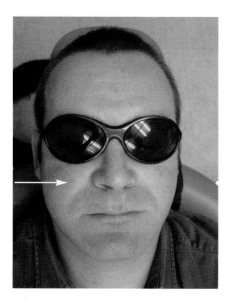

Figure 1.2

A patient with facial swelling (arrowed).

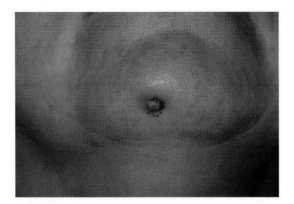

Figure 1.4

An external sinus tract on the chin that drained from the mandibular incisors.

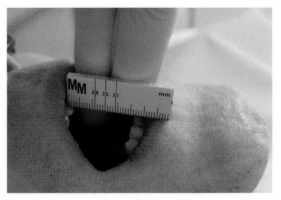

Figure 1.6

Sufficient opening is required to gain access to the teeth for endodontic treatment. Two fingers' width in the incisor region is perfectly adequate.

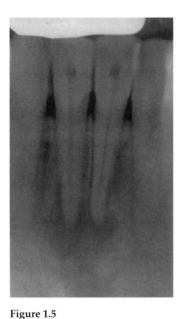

Figure 1.5

A paralleling radiograph of the mandibular incisors showed a periapical radiolucency. The central incisors were non-vital, and pus was draining through the external sinus tract.

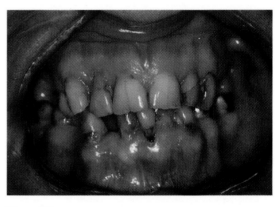

Figure 1.7

A neglected mouth. The patient will need advice on oral hygiene prior to endodontic treatment.

Grade I   1 mm Slight
Grade II   1–2 mm Moderate
Grade III > 2 mm and vertical Extensive

Mobility can result from trauma, root fractures, periodontal disease and gross root resorption. Sometimes a very slight (< 1 mm) degree of mobility may be normal. For instance, a tooth that has a horizontal root fracture in the middle third could be expected to have a degree of mobility, as would teeth under active orthodontic traction. Neither would necessarily require treatment purely because of the mobility.

and poorly finished? Is there obvious recurrent caries present (Figs. 1.8, 1.9)?

Tooth mobility: A suspect tooth can be moved gently by finger and thumb pressure; any horizontal mobility is then graded (Fig. 1.10).

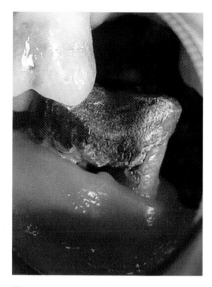

Figure 1.8

The overhanging restoration on the buccal surface of this mandibular molar has provided a site for plaque accumulation, and active caries is now present under the restoration.

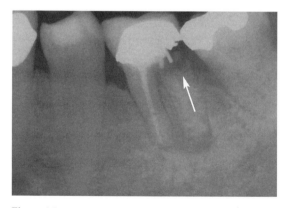

Figure 1.9

A radiograph showing advanced recurrent/root caries (arrowed). This tooth is probably unrestorable.

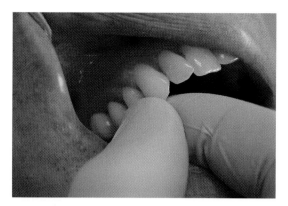

Figure 1.10

Testing tooth mobility by gently applying lateral forces between finger and thumb.

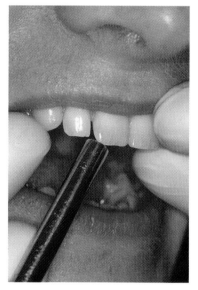

Figure 1.11

Gently percussing a tooth with a mirror handle may elicit the classical ringing sound that occurs with replacement resorption (ankylosis).

Tenderness to palpation: The tooth is moved vertically and side to side with finger pressure. Teeth with acute apical periodontitis will often be tender when palpated in this manner.

Percussion: Tapping a tooth with a mirror handle can help identify replacement resorption (ankylosis). A characteristic ringing sound is sometimes heard on percussion (Fig. 1.11).

Palpation of the buccal sulcus: Running a finger gently along the buccal sulcus will help elicit if there is any swelling or tenderness over the apex of an offending tooth (Figs. 1.12, 1.13).

Intraoral sinus tracts: These are usually seen on the attached buccal gingiva. The gingiva should be gently dried with a three-in-one syringe, and examined closely under good illumination (Figs. 1.14, 1.15). Running a finger along the mucosa may elicit a discharge from the sinus tract (Fig. 1.16). The tract exit may not always be adjacent to the offending tooth (Fig. 1.17). Sinus tracts exit less commonly on the palate (Fig. 1.18). When taking a radiograph for diagnosis it is useful to place a gutta percha point in the tract to identify the source of the problem (Figs. 1.19, 1.20).

Periodontal pocketing: Probing depths should be measured carefully with a periodontal probe. Ideally a probe with a tip of 0.5 mm should be used and pressure of no more than 25 g applied (light pressure!). Broad pockets are normally due to periodontal disease. A sudden increase in probing depth resulting in a narrow but deep pocket may indicate the position of a vertical root fracture or sinus tract lying within the periodontal ligament (Figs. 1.21–1.25).

Mobility of fixed prosthodontics: Inserting a probe under the pontic of a bridge and applying a pulling force can be used to test whether either abutment is loose (Fig. 1.26). The margins of full crown restorations can be tested with a probe (Figs. 1.27, 1.28).

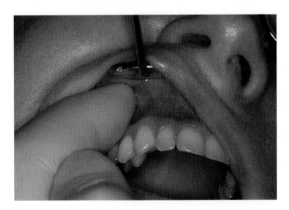

Figure 1.12

Palpating the buccal sulcus over the apices of the teeth, with a finger tip. Any tenderness or swelling is noted. Tenderness may be an indication of acute apical periodontitis.

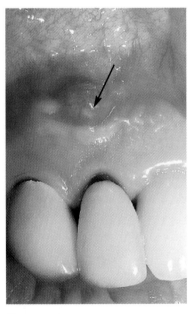

Figure 1.14

An intraoral sinus tract in the anterior region.

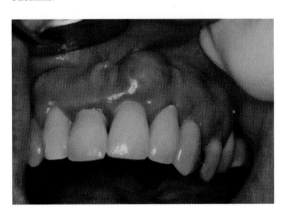

Figure 1.13

A buccal swelling in the anterior region. Some swellings may not be visible but can be palpated.

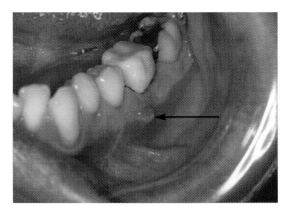

Figure 1.15

An intraoral sinus tract in the posterior region.

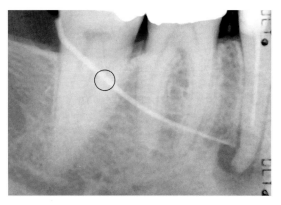

Figure 1.17

In this patient a sinus tract opposite the lower molar (indicated by ring) tracked along the mandible to the periapical abscess on the premolar. Sinus tracts do not always point adjacent to the offending tooth. Vitality testing and good radiological techniques are needed to identify the source of the problem.

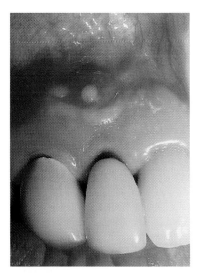

Figure 1.16

Pus discharging from the anterior sinus tract.

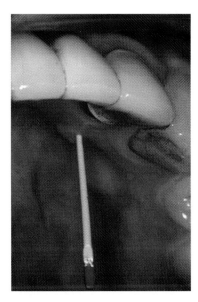

Figure 1.18

A palatal sinus tract in the anterior region.

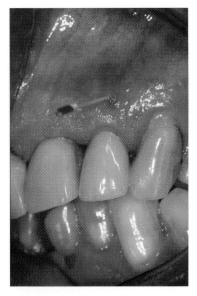

Figure 1.19

Placing a gutta percha point in a sinus tract to identify the source of the problem. This will not be painful, as the sinus tract is often epithelialized. Topical anaesthetic gel may occasionally be required.

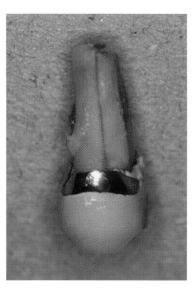

Figure 1.21

An extracted tooth with a vertical root fracture. In this case the tooth had fractured despite having been crowned.

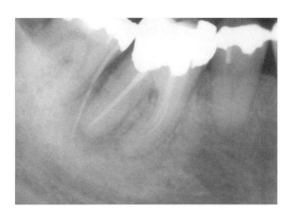

Figure 1.20

A radiograph of a gutta percha point inserted into a sinus tract adjacent to a mandibular molar.

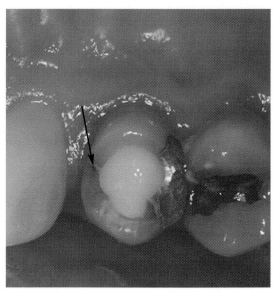

Figure 1.22

An occlusal view of a maxillary premolar that had fractured vertically in a mesial–occlusal–distal plane.

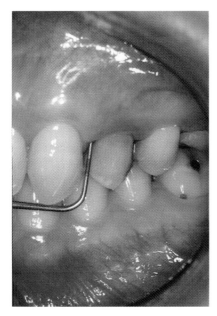

Figure 1.23

The maximum periodontal probing depth on the mesial aspect was 7 mm. The pocket shape was deep and narrow.

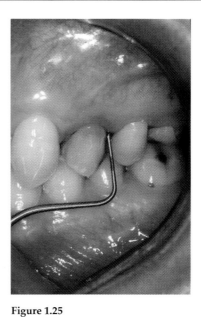

Figure 1.25

The probing depth of 7 mm on the distal aspect of the tooth directly opposite to that on the mesial aspect was indicative of a vertical root fracture.

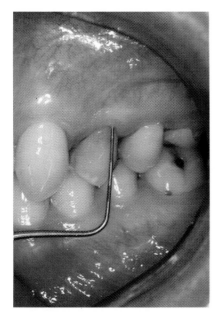

Figure 1.24

There were 1.0–1.5 mm probing depths buccally.

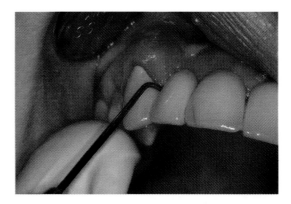

Figure 1.26

Inserting a probe under the pontic of a bridge to test for mobility.

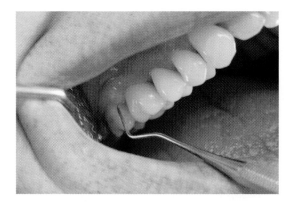

Figure 1.27

Testing for marginal deficiencies around a crown using a Briault probe.

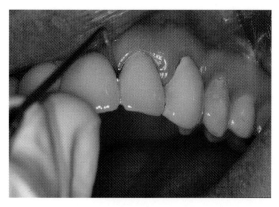

Figure 1.28

A DG16 probe (Hu Friedy, Chicago, IL, USA) can be used to test the margins of restorations.

SPECIAL TESTS

Pulp Testing

Pulp testing is used to assess whether a pulp is vital. Most methods test whether the nerve fibres within the pulp are able to conduct impulses. Laser Doppler flowmetry is still an experimental method of assessing the blood flow in the pulp.

The teeth adjacent to that with questionable pulp vitality and a contralateral tooth are often assessed to give a comparison. Sometimes more than one tooth may be the cause of a patient's symptoms. Teeth may be naturally sensitive or consistently record low responses to electric and thermal stimuli.

Thermal Tests

Cold. Cold can be applied to teeth in the form of an ice stick made using a needle cover, carbon dioxide snow, ethyl chloride on a pledget of cotton wool, cold water and rubber dam (Fig. 1.29). Blowing an air stream indiscriminately across the teeth from a three-in-one syringe is not a useful test of vitality, as it is impossible to isolate the air-stream to one tooth.

Heat. An electric heater-tip, rubber wheel, or hot gutta percha (Fig. 1.30) can be used. When using hot gutta percha it is wise to have local anaesthetic to hand and to cover the tooth surface with petroleum jelly to prevent the sticky rubber from adhering to the tooth (Figs. 1.31, 1.32). Isolating teeth individually with rubber dam and applying hot tap water in a syringe is an excellent method of testing individual teeth when diagnosis is difficult or if a patient describes the pain as being stimulated by a hot drink.

Electric Pulp Testing

Electric pulp testers use an electric current (AC or DC) to stimulate a response from the nerve tissue in the pulp. An example is the Analytic Technology pulp tester (Fig. 1.33). The unit switches on automatically when a circuit is made. The current at the tip is then increased by a microprocessor until the circuit is broken or maximum current is reached. A digital readout from 0 to 80 is given on an LED display. It is possible to increase or decrease the rate of electrical stimulus.

Method of use. The tooth to be tested is dried, to avoid short-circuiting through saliva into the periodontium. A tooth may also need to be isolated with strips of rubber dam between the contact points to prevent conduction through metallic restorations into adjacent teeth (Fig. 1.34). A small amount of conducting medium such as KY jelly or tooth-

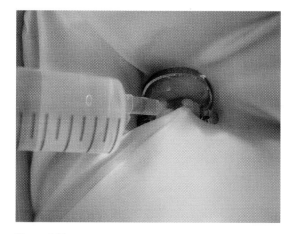

Figure 1.29

The tooth is isolated with rubber dam and immersed in cold water.

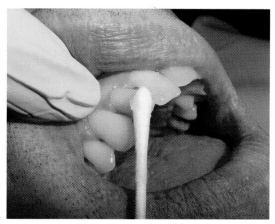

Figure 1.31

Vaseline is placed on the tooth surface to prevent the rubber sticking.

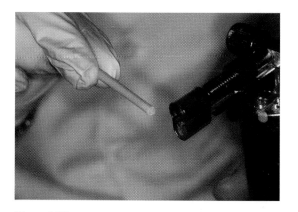

Figure 1.30

Hot gutta percha can be used to test a tooth for heat sensitivity.

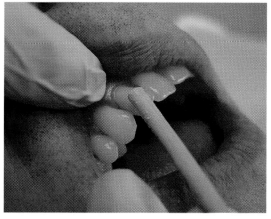

Figure 1.32

The heated gutta percha is placed on to the tooth.

paste is then applied to the tip of the pulp tester (Fig. 1.35). Mono-polar testers such as the Analytic Technology tester require the circuit to be completed by the operator or patient. Since the operator is wearing rubber gloves, the circuit will not be complete. The patient is asked to hold the metal handle of the instrument until a tingling sensation is felt in the tooth (Fig. 1.36); at this point the patient should let go and the stimulus will cease. A reading can be taken from the LED display.

It should be remembered that electric pulp testing does not give an indication of vascular health, which is especially important in traumatized immature teeth. It is possible to get a false positive reading via periodontal short-circuiting, and in multi-rooted teeth there may be varying degrees of vitality in separate roots.

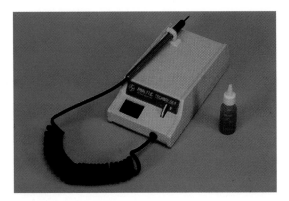

Figure 1.33

An electric pulp tester.

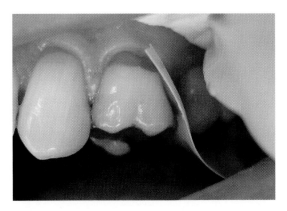

Figure 1.34

Adjacent teeth are sometimes isolated with rubber dam to prevent short-circuiting through metal restorations.

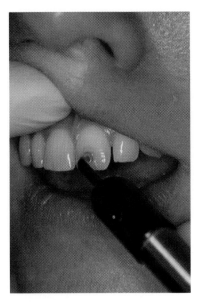

Figure 1.35

The tip of the electric pulp tester is coated in toothpaste to improve conductivity.

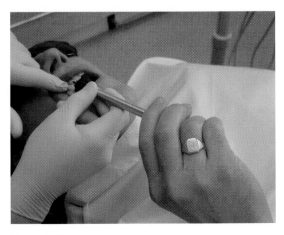

Figure 1.36

A circuit is made when the patient holds the metal handle.

Measurement of Blood Flow

Laser Doppler flowmetry. These units are not currently marketed for use in dental surgeries, but it may be possible to refer patients for Laser Doppler assessment at a teaching hospital. This method will give an indication of the vascular health of a pulp, and is particularly useful when assessing immature teeth that have been traumatized (Figs. 1.37, 1.38).

Other Methods

Local anaesthetic. Applying local anaesthetic as an intraligamental injection may help elicit the offending tooth. Teeth adjacent to the injection site may also be affected by the anaesthetic. This method could be used to identify whether a maxillary or mandibular tooth is the cause of referred pain.

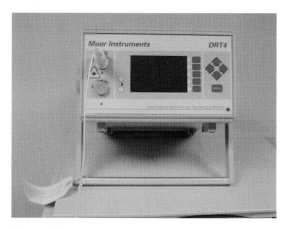

Figure 1.37

A Laser Doppler machine.

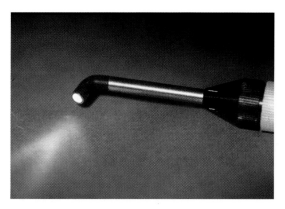

Figure 1.39

A fibre optic light for assessment of cracks.

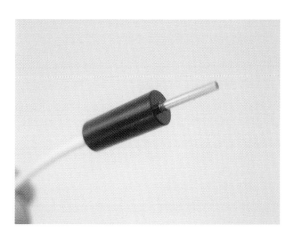

Figure 1.38

The Laser Doppler probe.

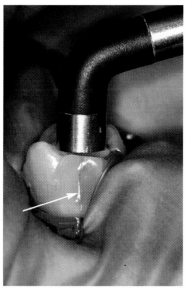

Figure 1.40

A tooth is illuminated to visualize a crack (arrowed).

Cutting a Test Cavity

As a last resort a cavity can be cut in the tooth with no local anaesthetic. This is not totally reliable, however, as sometimes partially necrotic pulps in teeth that require root canal treatment will respond to drilling. Cold coolant spray can also stimulate adjacent teeth.

Identifying Cracked Cusps

Teeth with cracked cusps are sometimes sensitive to thermal stimulation. Identifying the fractured cusp can be difficult, as the fracture line may not be visible to the naked eye.

Transillumination with a fibre optic light may highlight a crack (Figs. 1.39, 1.40).

A plastic 'Tooth Slooth' or wooden bite stick can be used to apply pressure to individual cusps on a tooth (Figs. 1.41, 1.42).

Asking a patient to bite on the corner of a folded sheet of rubber dam may elicit pain from a cracked cusp (Fig. 1.43).

RADIOGRAPHY

Accurate and predictable radiographic techniques are essential for endodontic diagnosis and treatment.

The X-ray Unit

The X-ray machine should comply with current ionizing radiation regulations. A tube voltage of 70 kV is ideally suited for intraoral radiography. The beam produced by the X-ray head is divergent, and must be filtered and collimated to produce a parallel source. Filtration is equivalent to 1.5 mm of aluminium for units up to 70 kV. Collimation

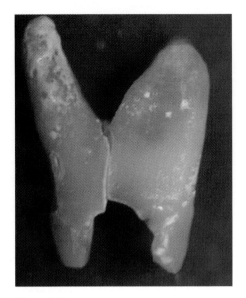

Figure 1.42

This tooth was completely fractured.

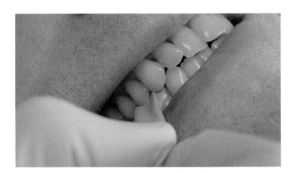

Figure 1.43

Biting on a rubber dam sheet may cause a cracked cusp to flex, aiding diagnosis.

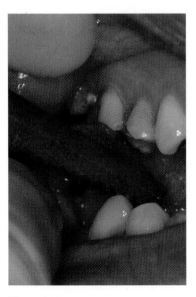

Figure 1.41

A Tooth Slooth being used to apply pressure to an individual cusp.

produces a beam that is no larger than 60 mm. A spacer cone allows correct alignment and correct distance from focal point to skin. This distance should be 200 mm for units operating at 70 kV. All X-ray units should have a warning light and sound to indicate when X-rays are being emitted.

Dose Reduction

It is important to keep all exposure to ionizing radiation as low as is reasonably achievable (ALARA). Whenever exposing the patient to X-radiation the clinician must assess the probability of obtaining useful information and ensure that it is maximized.

Physical methods of limiting and reducing the dose of radiation include:

- Only taking a radiograph when clinically essential
- Complying with Health and Safety regulations (including beam size and filtration)
- Using an X-ray unit with at least 70 kV output
- Using a film with the shortest exposure time feasible for the clinical condition.

All radiographic techniques should be made as accurate as possible. Avoiding the need to repeat films obviously reduces X-ray dose and maximizes the diagnostic value of each image.

Techniques Available

Radiographic films are probably the most widely used method in general dental practice. However, with increasing computerization digital radiography offers a new and exciting alternative.

Radiographic Film

The D-Speed radiographic film was used for many years, but has now been superseded by E-speed film, which gives excellent clarity of image with fine detail. Wet processing using fast-acting chemicals can produce a readable image for viewing in approximately 2 minutes.

Film speed. Film speed is a function of the number and size of the halide crystals in the emulsion. The larger the crystals the faster the film; but the quality of the image may suffer. In clinical situations the fastest film possible that will achieve the desired result should be used. For endodontic treatment there is no significant difference in the clarity of image when using D- or E-speed film. Most university dental schools now use E-speed film routinely.

Practical Points in General Radiographic Film Technique

Film Storage

Radiographic film should be stored in cool dry conditions (in a refrigerator) away from chemicals, especially mercury-containing compounds. The film packets should be stored well away from sources of ionizing radiation and boxed until required; this avoids films becoming damaged or bent. Films must not be bent, as otherwise an artefact will appear on the film.

Processing

Radiographic film can be developed manually or automatically. Processing involves two stages, development and fixing. To obtain good radiographic images careful quality control must be implemented and the physical conditions under which the films are processed must be tightly controlled and standardized.

Development

Development of the X-ray film should be carried out in complete darkness or filtered light, either in a darkroom or glove-box (Fig. 1.44). The entrance handles on such boxes should be replaced if they become worn or damaged, as this may allow light to penetrate the box. It is very important to mix developer solutions to the correct concentration according to the manufacturer's recommendations. Solutions must be replaced regularly and the containers

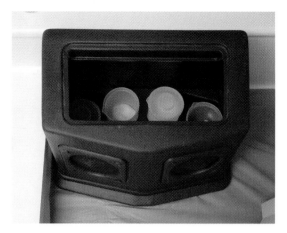

Figure 1.44

A hand-developing tank for radiographs.

washed thoroughly in clean water. Used developer solution should not be discarded in a surgery sink. Ready-mixed solutions are obviously easier to use, as they require no dilution. The temperature of developing solutions should be maintained at an optimum level (usually 20°C). To avoid fluctuations in temperature a glove-box should be positioned in the surgery away from direct sunlight, heaters or autoclaves. Increasing the temperature or extending development time will lead to dark unreadable films; if the solution is too cold or development time too short then a pale film will result.

Fixing

Fixing should be carried out in a dark environment or under filtered light. The concentration of the fixer solution is important for consistent results. Ideally the film should be fixed for twice the development time. It is possible however to view a film prematurely (working length estimation) before returning it to the fixing solution. Inadequate fixing results in a green/yellow discoloration that eventually turns brown.

Automatic Processors

Automatic development ensures that controlled standardized conditions for time and temperature of processing are maintained. The concentration of developer and fixer solutions is important for quality control and predictable results. The rollers and containers of automatic developers should be washed regularly to prevent build-up of chemicals.

Digital Radiography

Digital radiography is a relatively new development for dental use. It offers an exciting alternative to radiographic film.

Digital radiography consists of a sensor that creates an electrical signal that can be read by a computer and converted into a greyscale image. Most of the software necessary to produce digital radiographic images can be installed on computers routinely used in the dental surgery. Images can be enhanced in terms of contrast, filtering, brightness, subtraction and the addition of colours (Fig. 1.45).

Digital radiography can be direct or indirect. Direct systems have a sensor that is attached directly to the computer by a cable. This gives almost instantaneous images. Indirect systems use a laser reading device to scan the exposed sensor before generating an image.

The X-ray dose with digital systems is significantly reduced compared with E-speed film. Sensors tend to be expensive, fragile and relatively thick (5 mm). They have a life expectancy of approximately 400 000 doses (Figs. 1.46, 1.47).

Radiographic Techniques

Paralleling Technique

A paralleling technique is extremely useful in endodontics, and has several advantages over bisecting angle techniques.

Advantages of paralleling technique:

- Geometrically accurate image with little magnification. This enables the dentist to estimate root canal length prior to instrumentation.
- The periodontal membrane is well displayed. This is very useful in endodontics, as its widening or destruction is a good indicator of inflammation of endodontic origin.

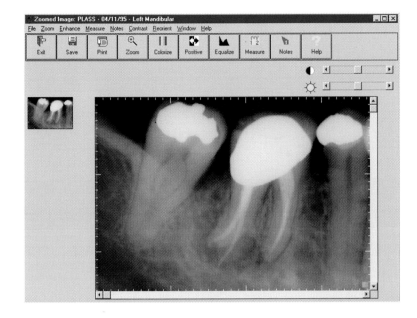

Figure 1.45

A digital image of a root-treated tooth taken with the Schick system (Schick Technologies Inc, Long Island City, NY, USA); the image manipulation effects can be seen at the top of the screen.

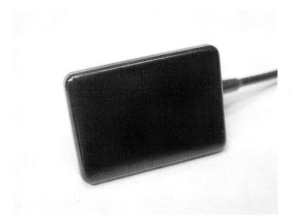

Figure 1.46

The Schick digital sensor.

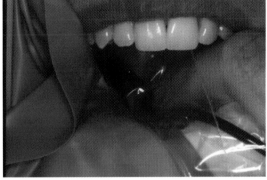

Figure 1.47

The sensor is placed in a polythene cover to prevent contamination and cross-infection. It can be held in position with the patient's finger, or in a special Rinn holder.

- There is minimal foreshortening or elongation of the periapical tissues.
- Coning off is reduced.
- If the same technique is used routinely then radiographs become almost reproducible. This is helpful for endodontic review.

Principles of the Paralleling Technique

The film packet is placed in a holder in the same plane as the long axis of the tooth. The tube-head is then aimed at a right angle to the tooth and film packet using an aiming device.

A holder should be used to help align the X-ray film and beam (Figs. 1.48–1.53).

The location of an area of radiolucency on the side of a root may be a sign of a lateral canal (Figs. 1.54, 1.55). Taking radiographs from a different horizontal angle can provide further information, displaying for instance extra root canals (Figs. 1.56, 1.57).

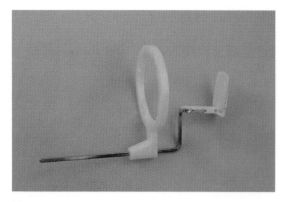

Figure 1.48

The Rinn holder paralleling device (Dentsply, Weybridge, Surrey, UK) for the anterior region.

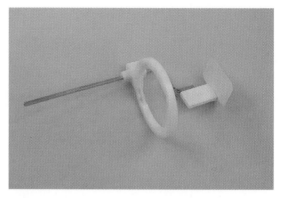

Figure 1.50

The Rinn holder paralleling device for the posterior region.

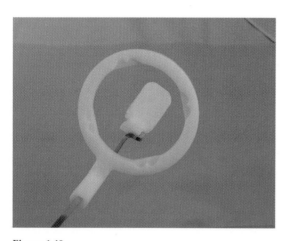

Figure 1.49

The anterior Rinn holder, beam aiming device.

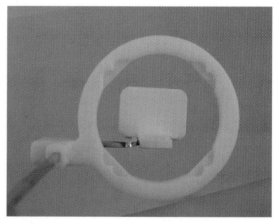

Figure 1.51

The posterior Rinn holder, beam aiming device.

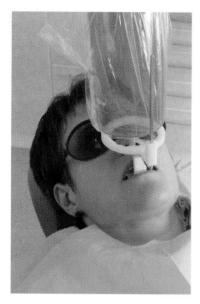

Figure 1.52

The anterior Rinn in use. The X-ray head is covered in a disposable polythene cover to prevent cross-infection.

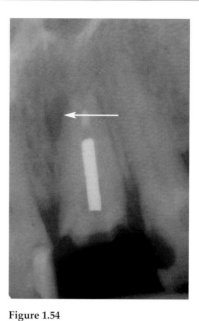

Figure 1.54

A lateral radiolucency may be an indication of a lateral canal.

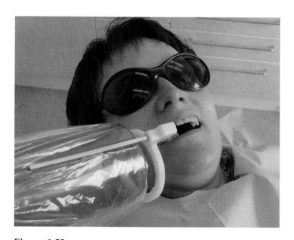

Figure 1.53

The posterior Rinn in use.

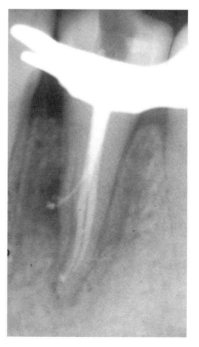

Figure 1.55

A lateral canal has been filled during obturation; it lies adjacent to a lateral radiolucency.

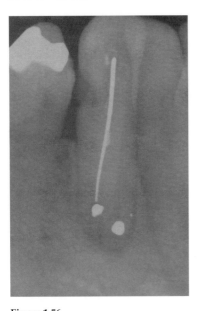

Figure 1.56

Rotating the cone produced a radiograph, showing an unfilled second canal.

The bisecting angle technique should really be reserved for cases in which it is impossible to fit a holder into the patient's mouth. It is also of value in locating a horizontal root fracture, especially if the fracture line lies in the plane of the X-ray beam (Fig. 1.58).

Retching. Using a topical local anaesthetic gel or spray can reduce retching. Distracting the patient by getting him/her to concentrate on gentle breathing can also help (Fig. 1.59).

Shallow palate. Placing a cotton wool roll on the occlusal surface of the teeth will help align the holder.

Edentulous spaces. So that the holder does not become tilted when the patient bites together a cotton wool roll may be used to support the bite plate (Figs. 1.60, 1.61).

Small mouth. It may not be physically possible to fit the holder plus standard film into a patient's mouth; in this case a small film can be used or a film can be held by artery forceps.

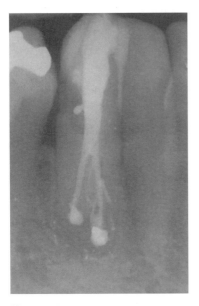

Figure 1.57

The completed obturation revealed an even more complicated root canal system.

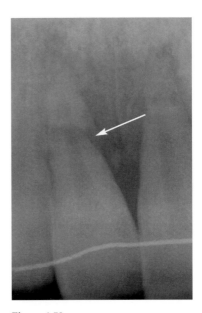

Figure 1.58

A bisecting angle film showed the horizontal root fracture (arrowed).

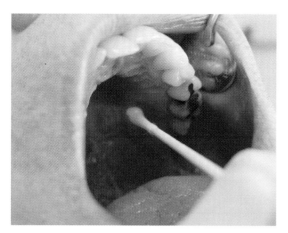

Figure 1.59

Application of topical anaesthetic gel to prevent retching.

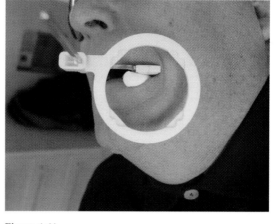

Figure 1.61

A cotton wool roll has been placed on the edentulous ridge to prevent the holder rotating.

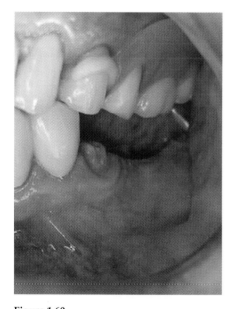

Figure 1.60

With an edentulous ridge the Rinn holder needs to be supported, as in this case, where a periapical radiograph is required of the mandibular premolar.

DIAGNOSIS

The clinician must listen to the patient's symptoms and summate the findings of several tests to come to a decision as to the likely cause of the patient's pain and whether the health of the pulp of the suspect tooth is affected. If two or more tests indicate that a tooth is non-vital and there is evidence of radiological change then the practitioner can be relatively confident of the diagnosis. If one is unsure or the findings are not conclusive a period of observation or referral would be appropriate (Figs. 1.62, 1.63).

Pulpal condition can clinically be classified under simple headings:

Normal pulp. The normal pulp gives a transient response to thermal tests and can be stimulated by electric pulp testing; it may also be sensitive to sweet and to acidic foods. The electric pulp tester may produce feelings varying from a tingling sensation to pain. Palpation and percussion do not cause pain. Radiologically there is a normal periodontal ligament space bounded by an intact lamina dura. The periodontal ligament space can appear increased in width over the apex of the palatal roots of upper molar teeth, owing to the magnifying effect of the air sinus.

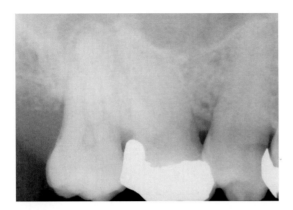

Figure 1.62

A diagnosis can be made after listening to the patient's symptoms and carrying out special tests. In this case the maxillary second molar appears to have an apical radiolucency. Special tests however reveal that the maxillary first molar is non-vital.

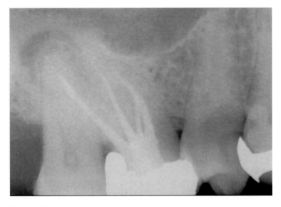

Figure 1.63

The completed root canal treatment shows that the roots of the maxillary molars are superimposed on the radiograph. A thorough and logical approach to diagnosis prevented incorrect treatment.

Reversible pulpitis. Pain induced by thermal stimuli tends to be of short duration (seconds rather than minutes), and does not radiate. Palpation and percussion do not stimulate pain. A filling may have been recently placed, or there may possibly be cracked cusps.

Irreversible pulpitis. Pain can be variable, from a spontaneous deep ache to total

absence. Initially pain can be referred, and is usually stimulated by thermal tests, when it lasts several minutes or hours. When pulpal inflammation reaches the apex, the tooth may become tender to bite on or respond to palpation. At this point there may be radiological changes apically.

Pulpal necrosis. If the entire pulp is necrotic then the tooth will fail to respond to thermal tests; however, in multi-rooted teeth the pulp in one root may remain vital, making diagnosis by thermal tests difficult. Radiologically, there are usually periapical changes (Fig. 1.64).

Periapically there may be:

Acute periapical inflammation. Classically the tooth becomes tender to bite on and is painful when palpated or percussed. On a radiograph there may be slight widening of the periodontal ligament apically.

Acute apical abscess. Pus forms around the apex, there may be swelling, and the tooth is tender to bite on. Severe infection may lead to pyrexia and a possible spread of infection along tissue planes. Radiolucency at the apex

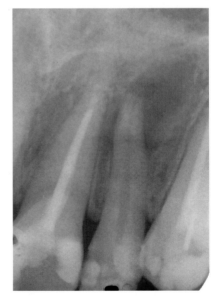

Figure 1.64

A radiograph of a tooth with pulpal necrosis; it was non-responsive to vitality testing.

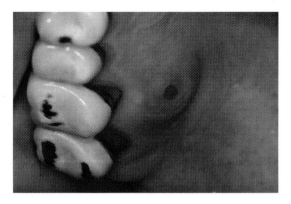

Figure 1.65

An acute abscess in the maxillary region has resulted in localized palatal swelling.

may not be readily observable in an acute abscess (Fig. 1.65).

Chronic apical periodontitis. This is frequently symptomless, but the tooth may occasionally produce symptoms. Radiologically there is a radiolucency at the apex of the tooth continuous with the periodontal ligament or adjacent to a lateral canal. A chronic lesion may become exacerbated and produce acute symptoms and signs.

FURTHER READING

Baumgartner JC, Heggers JP, Harrison JW (1976). The incidence of bacteraemias related to endodontic procedures. I Nonsurgical endodontics. *Journal of Endodontics* **2:** 135–140.

Baumgartner JC, Heggers JP, Harrison JW (1977). The incidence of bacteraemias related to endodontic procedures. II Surgical endodontics. *Journal of Endodontics* **3:** 399–402.

British Society for Antimicrobial Chemotherapy (1990). Prophylaxis of infective endocarditis. *Lancet* **355:** 88–89.

McGowan DA, Nair S, Macfarlane TW, Mackenzie D (1983). Prophylaxis of experimental endocarditis in rabbits using one or two doses of amoxycillin. *British Dental Journal* **155:** 88–90.

2 THREE-DIMENSIONAL ROOT CANAL ANATOMY

CONTENTS • **Introduction** • **Basic Anatomy of the Tooth and Surrounding Structures** • **Individual Tooth Anatomy** • **Further Reading**

INTRODUCTION

A clear understanding of pulp anatomy and the variations that occur in it are essential if effective cleaning, shaping and obturation of the pulp space are to be achieved. Many problems that occur during root canal treatment result from poor knowledge of this anatomy: missed canals, perforation of the pulp floor or canal transportation. If the clinician can imagine a three-dimensional picture of the root canal system prior to instrumentation then iatrogenic errors are less likely to occur. The practitioner should be aware of how many canals to expect, their location, length and relationship to each other.

BASIC ANATOMY OF THE TOOTH AND SURROUNDING STRUCTURES

The Pulp

The pulp is connective tissue, consisting mainly of odontoblasts and fibroblasts. Glycosaminoglycans form the ground substance, which is penetrated with collagen fibres. A main neurovascular bundle enters the foramen at the apex of the tooth. Arterioles are the largest afferent vessels found in the pulp and pass towards the crown along the axis of the tooth, giving off branches that terminate in the subodontoblastic capillary plexus. There are interconnections known as anastomoses between the venules and arterioles. This feature allows the re-routing of blood flow, preventing the build-up of unsustainable pressure in the enclosed pulp environment. The pulp is richly innervated, containing myelinated Aδ and Aβ fibres (fast-conducting) and unmyelinated C fibres (slow-conducting). Mild, transient, low-threshold noxious stimuli (mechanical, thermal, chemical or electrical) activate fast-conducting Aδ fibres, while high-threshold, long-duration or inflammatory stimuli activate C fibre neurones. The C fibres give rise to the sensation of poorly localized, throbbing and aching pain; stimulation does not occur until the pulp tissue is damaged. Myelinated Aβ fibres have the most rapid conduction velocity; they may be involved in regulating masticatory forces and could also provide innervation for dentine sensitivity. Autonomic fibres of the sympathetic system control the microcirculation. The nerve fibres terminate in the pulp dentine border area as the plexus of Raschkow; individual axons then branch into terminal filaments that enter some dentine tubules. The pulp is enclosed in a space surrounded by dentine, with which it forms the *pulp dentine complex*.

Dentine

Dentine is produced by odontoblasts and forms the bulk of the mineralized portion of the tooth. This dentine is covered by enamel on the crown of the tooth, and cementum over the root surface. Embryonically dentine and pulp are both derived from the dental papilla and have a close relationship in structure, function and development. Dentine tubules radiate from the pulp towards the enamel and cementum. There are approximately 57 000 tubules per mm^2 in the dentine adjacent to the pulp, with an average diameter of approximately 3 µm, making 80% of the volume of the tissue. At the amelo-dentine junction there are approximately 8000 tubules per mm^2, with diameters of about 1 µm, or 4% of the total volume. In the crown the tubules follow an S-shaped curve. Odontoblast cell bodies are separated from the mineralized dentine by the unmineralized predentine layer, which is 15 µm thick. The odontoblasts are arranged in a single layer, and have processes that extend into the tubules of the dentine. The processes extend for some distance within the tubules and have branches. In the inner dentine there are unmyelinated nerve terminals spiralling around some odontoblast processes.

Primary dentine is laid down before the tooth is fully formed. Following this, regular secondary dentine is formed at a much slower rate. As this is laid down the pulp chamber becomes smaller with age; this can make endodontic treatment more difficult in elderly patients. Peritubular dentine is also formed with age, and lines the dentine tubules. The production of dentine can be increased by stimuli such as caries, attrition and abrasion. Tubules can become completely occluded, giving rise to sclerotic dentine. The odontoblasts lay down irritation dentine at a fast rate as a defence mechanism, and this can on occasions virtually occlude the pulp space.

Root Canals (Figs. 2.1–2.4)

The root canals are continuous with the pulp chamber. The root canal space is often complex, with canals that divide and rejoin, fins, deltas and lateral canals. It is more like a subterranean cave formation, with interconnecting chambers carved out of limestone, than a simple mine shaft. For this reason many clinicians now refer to the root canal as a system, to convey this complexity. Attempts have been made to classify the different varieties of canal configuration, but most are two-dimensional and not always helpful clinically.

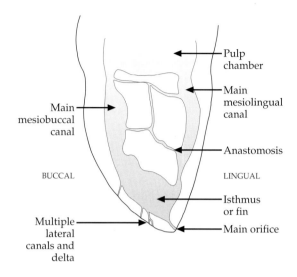

Figure 2.1

Root canal anatomy

The mesial root of a mandibular first molar in buccal-lingual section, showing various types of complex anatomy.

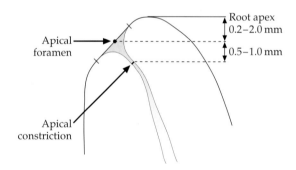

Figure 2.2

The apical constriction

The average distance between the apical foramen and the most apical part of the root is 0.2–2.0 mm. The constriction can be 0.5–1.0 mm from the apical foramen.

Root canals are generally broader buccolingually; but unless the tooth is severely rotated this is not apparent radiologically. This is of relevance because mechanical instrumentation will rarely be effective on all surfaces of a canal with an oval cross-section. During root development the root sheath

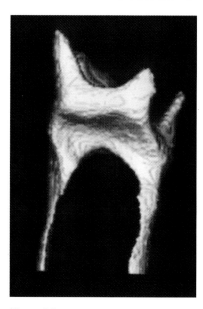

Figure 2.3

A microcomputed tomographic (MCT) scan of the pulp chamber of a mandibular second molar. Four pulp horns can be clearly seen. The orifices to the canals are funnel-like and extend into the canals, which are narrow mesiodistally.

folds, producing interconnections that persist between the periodontal and pulpal tissues in the fully developed tooth. In the apical region this can create a delta of tributaries projecting from the main canal that exit the root as multiple foramina. The root canal becomes narrowest approximately 1.0–1.5 mm from the main foramen. This point is known as the apical constriction, and lies just prior to the layer of cementum that covers the root. The position of such a constriction is variable and not visible on a radiograph, and can be completely destroyed by inflammatory resorption. It is therefore impossible for clinicians to estimate this point by tactile methods alone, and this confirms the need for other methods, for example an apex locator and a radiograph, to try to estimate root canal length during endodontic treatment. A tooth may have several apical, accessory and lateral canals. Lateral canals are also present in the furcation region of some molar teeth. The presence of a lateral canal can sometimes be seen radiologically when the root canal system is infected, because breakdown products within the lateral canal cause inflammatory responses in the periradicular tissues, leading to a lateral radiolucency on the radiograph. The integrity of the existing apical constriction should be maintained during root canal preparation. Studies have shown that the average distance

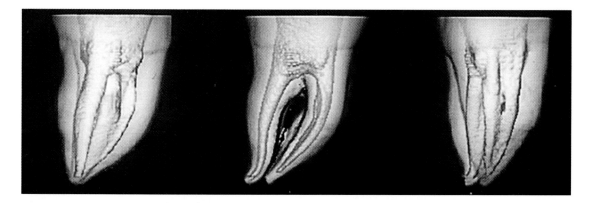

Figure 2.4

A MCT scan of a mandibular first molar; the three pictures show the tooth rotated through 60 degrees. An access cavity has been cut and the root canals prepared. The root canal system is complex, and a fin can be seen between the two mesial canals.

between the apical foramen and the most apical part of the root is variable over 0.2–2.0 mm, and furthermore the constriction can be 0.5–1.0 mm from the apical foramen. This gives credence to preparation techniques that maintain a small apical instrument size in order to cause as little damage to this region as possible.

Cementum

Cementum covers the radicular dentine. Acellular cementum does not contain cementocyte cell bodies, and forms the impervious innermost layer of cementum covering the root surface. The cementum forms a connection between the periodontal ligament and the tooth.

Periodontal Ligament (Fig. 2.5)

The periodontal ligament is a fibrous connective tissue. Fibres run in specific groups: gingival, transeptal, alveolar crest, horizontal, oblique and apical. There are many cells found in the periodontal ligament space: fibroblasts, occasionally defence cells, and the cell rests of Malassez. The cell rests are formed from the root sheath of Hertwig, which becomes perforated like a fishnet stocking. The periodontal ligament is supplied with nutrients from arterioles that enter near the apex of the root, and from the lateral walls of the alveolar socket. Venules drain blood in the opposite direction. Nerves provide sensory information for touch, pain and pressure, allowing proprioception during mastication. The periodontal ligament provides the visco-elastic connection between the tooth and the alveolar bone.

Alveolar Bone

Alveolar bone is the mineralized tissue that surrounds the teeth in the jaws. It is continuously formed by osteoblasts, and when these cells become incorporated in the tissue they are called osteocytes. Bone resorption is continuous and is carried out by osteoclasts, which lie in Howship's lacunae. There are two types of bone: cortical and cancellous. The spaces between the trabeculae of spongy bone may be filled with marrow.

INDIVIDUAL TOOTH ANATOMY (Table 2.1)

Maxillary Central Incisor (Figs. 2.6, 2.7)

The average length of maxillary central incisors is 22.5 mm. They normally have a single root and a single canal with an average volume of $12.4\,mm^3$ when fully formed. Mesiodistally the pulp chamber follows the general outline of the crown. It is widest at the most coronal level and has pulp horns. In young patients there may be three pulp horns that correspond to enamel mammelons on the incisal edge. Buccopalatally the pulp chamber is narrow as it transforms into the root canal with a constriction just apical to the cervix. In

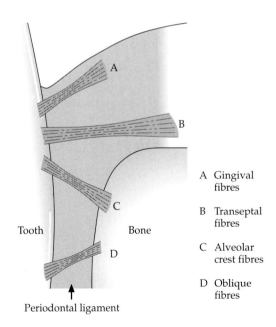

A Gingival fibres

B Transeptal fibres

C Alveolar crest fibres

D Oblique fibres

Tooth   Bone

Periodontal ligament

Figure 2.5

Periodontal fibres.

Table 2.1 *Three-dimensional root canal anatomy*

Tooth	Average length (mm)	Minimum length (mm)	Maximum length (mm)	Number of canals	Average mature pulp volume (mm^3)
Maxilla					
1	22.5	18.0	22.5	1	12.4 ± 3.3
2	21.0	17.0	26.0	1	11.4 ± 4.6
3	26.5	20.0	32.0	1	14.7 ± 4.8
4	21.0	17.0	22.5	1 2 (66%)	18.2 ± 5.1
5	21.5	16.0	27.0	1	16.5 ± 4.2
6	21.0	17.0	24.0	3 4 (66%)	68.2 ± 21.4
7	20.0	16.0	24.0	3	44.3 ± 29.7
8	—	—	—	Variable	—
Mandible					
1	21.0	16.0	24.0	1 2 (40%)	6.1 ± 2.5
2	21.0	18.0	27.0	1 2 (40%)	7.1 ± 2.1
3	22.5	18.0	32.5	1 2 (14%)	14.2 ± 5.4
4	21.5	18.0	26.0	1 2 (33%) 3 (32%)	14.9 ± 5.7
5	22.5	18.0	26.0	1 2 (11%)	14.9 ± 6.3
6	21.0	18.0	24.0	3 4 (31%)	52.4 ± 8.5
7	20.0	18.0	22.0	2 3 'C' shaped	32.9 ± 8.4
8	—	—	—	Variable	—

Modified from Black (1897) and Fanibunda (1986)

three dimensions it has a shape somewhat similar to a baseball glove. The constriction cannot always be seen radiologically. Coronally, the root canal is wider buccopalatally, with an oval cross-sectional shape; it becomes circular at the apex. With age the roof of the pulp chamber recedes and the canal appears much narrower on clinical radiographs. This can be deceptive, because buccopalatally the canal may still be much wider, and in three dimensions the canal is more ribbon-shaped.

Clinical Points

- In a young patient a pulp horn can be exposed following a relatively small fracture of an incisal corner. If a child presents with a crown fracture then the dentine in this region should be protected to prevent bacterial ingress into the pulp chamber.
- Placing the access cavity too far palatally makes straight-line access impossible. Transportation and ledging of the root canal will be more likely to occur on the buccal surfaces of the root canal. It may be

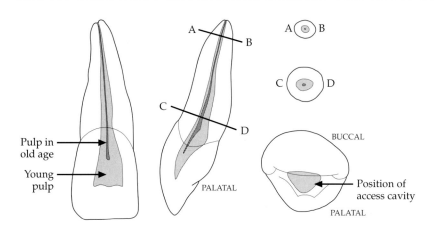

Pulp in old age

Young pulp

PALATAL

BUCCAL

Position of access cavity

PALATAL

Figure 2.6

Maxillary central incisor.

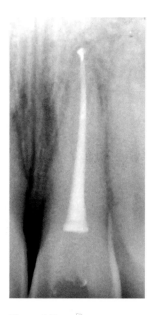

Figure 2.7

A maxillary central incisor.

necessary to extend the access cavity towards the incisal edge.
- Palatal tooth tissue should be conserved, as this is important for retention of full coverage restorations should they be necessary.
- In order to clean a ribbon-shaped canal effectively the operator relies on irrigant penetrating areas that the files do not reach.

Maxillary Lateral Incisor (Figs. 2.8, 2.9)

Lateral incisor teeth are generally shorter than maxillary central incisors, and have an average length of 21 mm. There is usually only one canal, with an average mature pulp space volume of 11.4 mm^3. Developmental anomalies such as *dens invaginatus* are sometimes seen. Pulp horns are more marked than in central incisors, and the incisal outline of the pulp chamber tends to be more rounded than that of central incisors. The apical region of the root canal is often curved in a palatal direction.

Clinical Points

- The palatal curvature of the apical region is rarely seen radiologically. The curvature can be abrupt, and is easily ledged during root canal preparation. This is a common finding in lateral incisors where the root filling is short of the apex. Precurving files or using a balanced force technique will help to avoid this.
- The cervical constriction may need to be removed during coronal flaring to produce a smooth progression from pulp chamber to root canal.
- In surgical endodontic treatment an apical curvature can complicate resection and root-end cavity preparation.

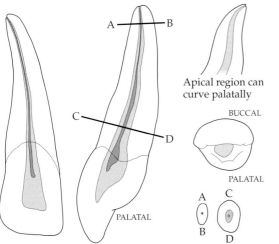

Apical region can curve palatally

Figure 2.8

Maxillary lateral incisor.

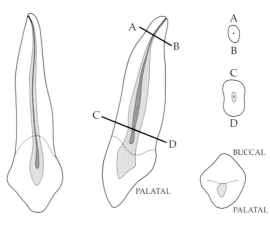

Figure 2.10

Maxillary canine.

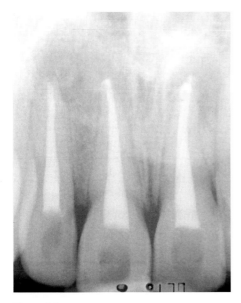

Figure 2.9

These young maxillary incisors have wide pulp chambers.

Maxillary Canine (Fig. 2.10)

This is usually the longest tooth, with an average length of 26.5 mm. It rarely has more than one root canal. The pulp chamber tends to be narrow, and pointed incisally. There can be a constriction at the cervix. The pulp space has an average mature volume of 14.7 mm^3 and is wider buccopalatally, along the length of the root. The root canal is, therefore, oval, in cross-section and only becomes circular in the apical third. The root apex is often tapered and thin, and may occasionally curve rather abruptly in a buccal or palatal direction.

Clinical Points

- When preparing long, sclerosed root canals great care must be taken to avoid blocking the root canal. Irrigation is imperative, and a lubricant may be helpful.
- The cervical constriction often needs to be shaped during coronal flaring to produce a smooth taper from the access cavity into the main body of the root canal.
- Surgical access to the apical region can be difficult when these teeth are particularly long.

Maxillary First Premolar (Figs. 2.11–2.14)

This tooth normally has two roots and two canals; however, single-rooted maxillary first premolars occur in one-third of Caucasians. In Mongoloids this figure is in excess of two-

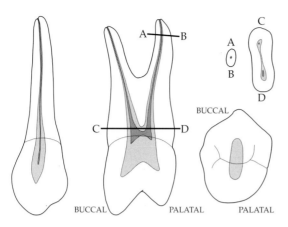

Figure 2.11

Maxillary first premolar.

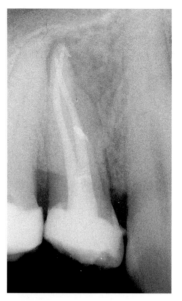

Figure 2.13

A maxillary first premolar with two canals.

thirds. Maxillary first premolars with three roots have been reported; and these usually show a similar morphological arrangement to maxillary molars. Generally, the average length of the first premolar is 21 mm and the average pulp volume is 18.2 mm^3. The pulp chamber is wider buccopalatally, with two pulp horns. The chamber appears much narrower on radiographs. Root canal orifices lie buccally and palatally. With age secondary dentine is deposited on the roof of the pulp chamber. The root canals are usually fairly straight, divergent and round in cross-section.

Clinical Points

- Taking radiographs from an angle can separate the root canals and avoid superimposition. The X-ray cone is usually rotated anteriorly. A common reason for unsuccessful root canal treatment in maxillary first premolars is a failure to locate both canals.

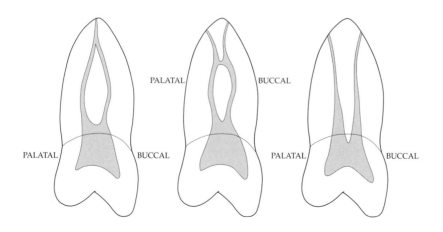

Figure 2.12

Maxillary first premolar root canal configurations.

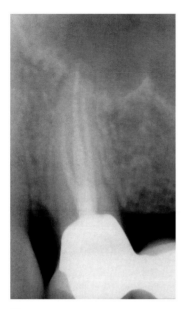

Figure 2.14

A maxillary first premolar with three canals; these are orientated in a similar manner to the maxillary first molar.

- It is sometimes possible to mistake the pulp horns for the orifices of the canals. Measurement from the preoperative radiograph and good intraoral illumination as well as magnification should avoid this mistake.
- The buccal root often has a palatal groove, which can be perforated during instrumentation if the coronal part of the root canal is over-flared.
- Surgically the palatal root may be difficult to reach. This may not necessarily be obvious on a preoperative radiograph, and surgical endodontics on maxillary first premolars should not be undertaken lightly for many reasons.

Maxillary Second Premolar (Figs. 2.15, 2.16)

The maxillary second premolar usually has one root and a single canal, but the shape of

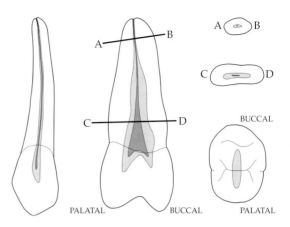

Figure 2.15

Maxillary second premolar.

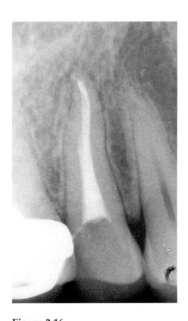

Figure 2.16

In this maxillary second premolar the single root canal has a 'ribbon-like' shape.

the canal system is variable. There may be a single canal along the entire length of the root. A single orifice may divide into two canals and emerge apically as one or two canals. Rarely there may be two or three separate canals branching from a single orifice. The average length of the maxillary second premolar is

21.5 mm and the average pulp volume 16.5 mm³. The pulp chamber is wide buccopalatally and has two well-defined pulp horns. The canal is also usually wider buccopalatally. The canal system therefore should be thought of as ribbon-like. This ribbon-like canal may be tortuous, becoming circular in cross-section only in the apical 2–3 mm. The root is generally straight; however, with age the roof of the pulp chamber recedes.

Clinical Points

- The canal can look deceptively thin on radiographs, but is ribbon-like in cross-section. This space can be difficult to clean and obturate effectively.
- It is sometimes possible to mistake the pulp horns for the canal orifice.

Maxillary First Molar (Figs. 2.17–2.23)

The maxillary first molar is generally three-rooted, with three or four canals. The mesiobuccal root contains two canals in approximately 60% of cases. The two canals in the mesiobuccal root are usually closely interconnected and sometimes merge into one canal or can be joined by a fin. The average length of this tooth is 21 mm, and the average pulpal volume 68.2 mm³. The bulk of the pulp

chamber lies mesial to the oblique ridge across the occlusal surface of the tooth. The palatal root orifice is usually the largest and easiest to locate, and appears funnel-like in the floor of the pulp chamber. The distobuccal canal orifice is located more palatally than the main mesiobuccal canal. The minor mesiobuccal canal (MB2) is located on a line between the palatal canal orifice and the main mesiobuccal canal orifice. The palatal root canal has a rounded triangular cross-section coronally and becomes circular apically. The canal may curve buccally in the apical 3–5 mm. The distobuccal canal tends to be round in cross-section and is normally the shortest canal; it may curve abruptly at the apex. The main mesiobuccal canal often exits the pulp chamber in a mesial direction but then curves distopalatally. The mesial canals are often joined by an isthmus, especially in the apical 3–5 mm. This makes the canal ribbon-shaped. The minor mesiobuccal canal can be extremely fine and tortuous. With age all the canals become narrower, and secondary dentine is laid down on the pulp chamber roof. A lip of dentine often obscures the minor mesiobuccal canal.

Clinical Points

- The pulp chamber lies mesial to the oblique ridge across the occlusal surface of the tooth. An access cavity should be cut

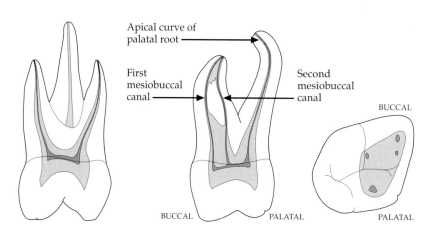

Apical curve of palatal root

First mesiobuccal canal

Second mesiobuccal canal

BUCCAL

BUCCAL   PALATAL   PALATAL

Figure 2.17

Maxillary first molar.

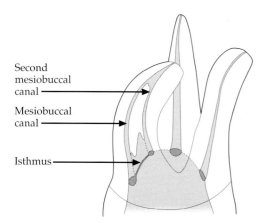

Second mesiobuccal canal

Mesiobuccal canal

Isthmus

Figure 2.18

The maxillary first molar.

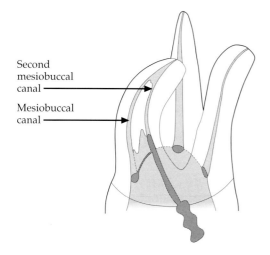

Second mesiobuccal canal

Mesiobuccal canal

Figure 2.19

Gaining access to the second mesiobuccal canal can best be achieved from a posterior aspect, aiming the file tip mesially.

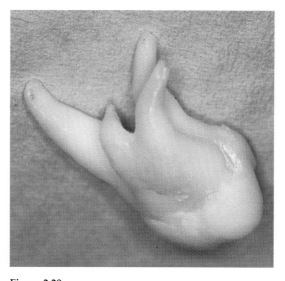

Figure 2.20

The maxillary first molar can have very curved mesiobuccal roots.

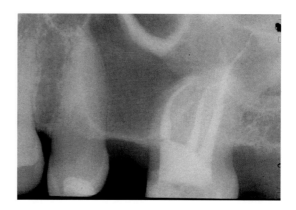

Figure 2.21

A maxillary first molar with three canals.

mesial to the oblique ridge, and will usually be triangular in shape.
- Secondary dentine and irritation dentine are laid down on the roof of the pulp chamber. Care should be taken, by study of the preoperative radiograph, to avoid perforation of the pulp floor when the two are in close proximity.
- As a consequence of dental caries, canal orifices may be considerably obstructed by irritation dentine, and therefore care is required in their identification.
- The mesiobuccal canals can curve severely, and the degree of curvature may not always be apparent radiologically. Care must be taken during preparation to avoid procedural errors.
- The orifice of the minor mesiobuccal canal

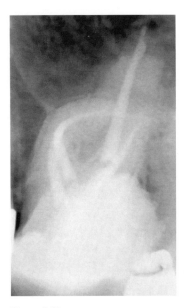

Figure 2.22

The mesiobuccal canals are often curved, and can be difficult to negotiate.

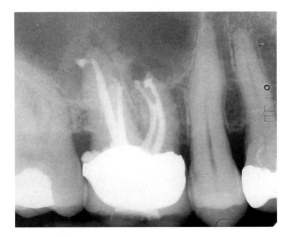

Figure 2.23

In this case the two mesiobuccal canals are separate, but there is an interconnection in the mid-third of the root.

can usually be detected under a lip of dentine on the mesial wall of the pulp chamber.
- The minor mesiobuccal canal should be approached from a distopalatal angle (i.e. aiming from the patient's throat), as the initial canal curvature is often mesial.
- The palatal root may have a buccal curvature that can be abrupt and not visible on a radiograph. Care should be taken to avoid instrumentation errors.
- There is often an isthmus between the mesiobuccal canals. Failure to clean this may result in failure of treatment.
- Surgical access to the first molar is extremely difficult.

Maxillary Second Molar (Fig. 2.24)

This tooth is similar to the maxillary first molar. The roots tend to be less divergent and may be fused. The average tooth length is 20 mm and average pulp canal volume is 44.3 mm^3. Sometimes with fusion of the roots the pulp chamber becomes distorted and elongated buccopalatally. The root canal orifices may be arranged almost in a line, with those of the mesiobuccal and distobuccal canals being very close.

Maxillary Third Molar

The maxillary third molar displays great variability in pulp chamber and root canal shape. There may be one, two or three canals.

Mandibular Incisors (Figs. 2.25–2.28)

Both the mandibular central and lateral incisors have an average length of 21 mm. The pulp chamber is similar in form to that of the maxillary incisors, being pointed incisally with three pulp horns. The pulp chamber is oval in cross-section. Average pulp volumes are 6.1 mm^3 for mature mandibular central incisors and 7.1 mm^3 for lateral incisors. Different root canal formations have been demonstrated. There may be one canal that extends from pulp chamber to apex. Sometimes two canals originate from the pulp chamber and merge apically. Two separate canals are found in some instances. The inci-

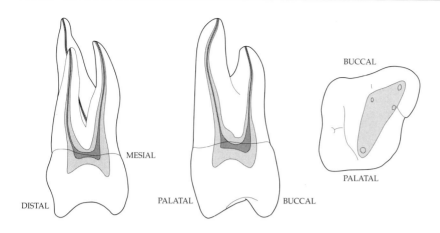

Figure 2.24

Maxillary second molar.

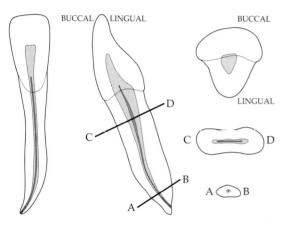

Figure 2.25

Mandibular incisors.

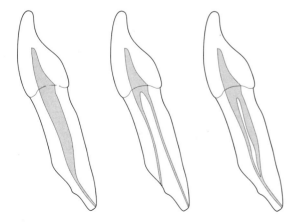

Figure 2.26

Mandibular incisor canal configurations.

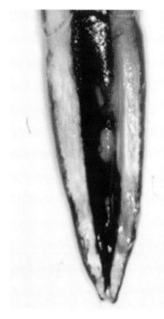

Figure 2.27

A cleared mandibular incisor. The root canal space is wider buccolingually than mesiodistally.

dence of cases of two canals can be as high as 41%. The canals are wider buccolingually than mesiodistally.

Clinical Points

- The presence of two canals may be missed on a preoperative radiograph if the canals are superimposed.

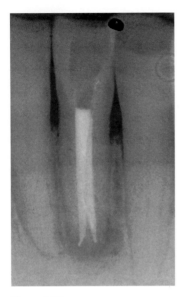

Figure 2.28

A mandibular incisor with two canals.

- The lingual canal is most often missed in teeth with two canals because the access cavity, if placed too far lingually, restricts straight-line access.
- It is easy to over-prepare the root canals of mandibular incisors, as the roots are fine. There is also a groove running down the length of the root on the mesial and distal surfaces. Over-preparation will weaken the tooth unnecessarily, and may result in strip perforation.
- The apices of mandibular incisors are often reclined lingually, and access for endodontic surgery can be extremely difficult.

Mandibular Canine (Figs. 2.29, 2.30)

This tooth bears a striking resemblance to the maxillary canine, but is smaller, with an average length of 22.5 mm and an average mature pulp volume of 14.2 mm³. This tooth usually has one root and one canal, but can occasionally have two (14%). The pulp chamber is pointed coronally, and there can be a cervical constriction. Coronally the root canal is oval in cross-section, becoming round in the apical region.

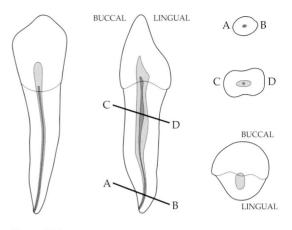

Figure 2.29

Mandibular canine.

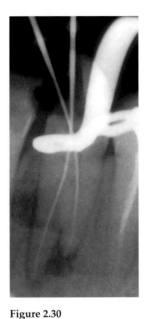

Figure 2.30

This mandibular canine has two canals.

Clinical Point

- In older patients where there has been significant deposition of secondary dentine it may be necessary to incorporate the incisal edge into the access cavity to ensure straight-line access and locate the root canal.

Mandibular First Premolar (Figs. 2.31, 2.32)

This tooth usually has one root and one canal. However a second canal has been identified in up to a third of teeth, and three canals occasionally. The pulp chamber has two pulp horns, the buccal horn being most prominent. In cross-section the chamber is oval, with the greatest dimension buccolingually. The average root length is 21.5 mm and the average mature pulp volume 14.9 mm^3. Root canal cross-sections tend to be oval until the most apical extents, where they become round.

Clinical Points

- The access cavity in these teeth may have to extend on to the cusp tip, in order to gain straight-line access.
- The lingual canal when present is notoriously difficult to instrument. Access can usually be gained by running a fine instrument down the lingual wall of the main buccal canal until the orifice is located; this may be several millimetres down the canal.
- Surgical access to the apex of the mandibular first premolar is often complicated by the proximity of the mental nerve.

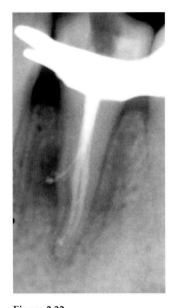

Figure 2.32

A mandibular first premolar with two diverging canals. There is an interconnection in the apical third and a long lateral canal.

Mandibular Second Premolar (Fig. 2.33)

This tooth usually has one root and one canal. Up to 11% of teeth have a second canal. The pulp chamber has two pulp horns; the lingual horn is more prominent

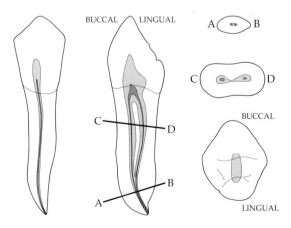

Figure 2.31

Mandibular first premolar.

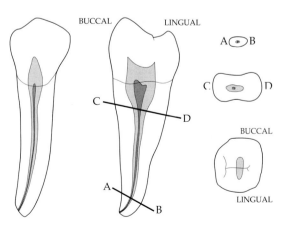

Figure 2.33

Mandibular second premolar.

than in the mandibular first premolar. In cross-section the pulp chamber is oval, with the greatest dimension buccolingually. The average root length is 22.5 mm and the average mature pulp volume 14.9 mm^3. Root canal cross-sections tend to be oval coronally and round apically.

Clinical Points

Similar to mandibular first premolar.

Mandibular First Molar (Figs. 2.34–2.38)

This tooth usually has two roots, which have average lengths of 21 mm and an average mature pulp volume of 52.4 mm^3. The pulp chamber is quadrilateral in cross-section at the level of the pulp floor and is wider mesially than distally. There may be four or five pulp horns. The distal root tends to be more rounded than the mesial root, which has a kidney bean shape in cross-section at the mid-third. There are usually two canals in the mesial roots and one in the distal. Approximately a third of distal roots contain two canals. The two mesial canals merge in approximately 45% of cases to a single foramen. The single distal canal is ribbon-shaped and has its largest dimension buccolingually. The mesiobuccal canal is generally curved, and often exits the pulp chamber in a mesial direction, while the mesiolingual canal tends

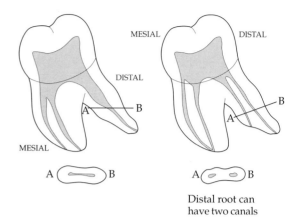

Distal root can have two canals

Figure 2.35

Mandibular first molar.

to be straighter. There is nearly always an isthmus between the two mesial canals in the apical third.

Clinical Points

- The mesial canals are small, and should not be over-enlarged to avoid procedural errors such as transportation.
- The mesial canals are curved in a mesiodistal and a buccolingual direction. The curved furcation wall is particularly vulnerable to perforation during root canal preparation by filing, as instruments straighten in the canal.

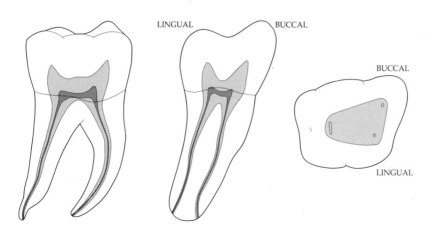

Figure 2.34

Mandibular first molar.

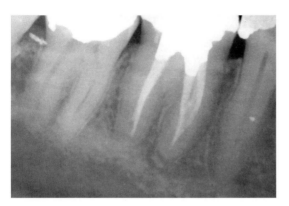

Figure 2.36

The mandibular first molar with three canals. A fin or isthmus often interconnects the mesial canals. There are lateral canals projecting from the main distal canal.

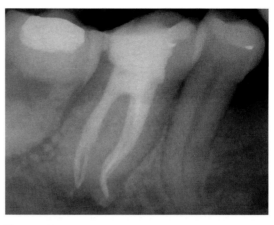

Figure 2.38

In this mandibular molar the canals are highly curved and there are many interconnections. The distal canal divides into two canals in the apical third.

- Root-end surgery on the mandibular first molar is complicated. Access is often difficult, and the root ends can be in close proximity to the inferior dental nerve and mental nerve.

Mandibular Second Molar (Fig. 2.39)

In Caucasians the mandibular second molar is similar to the mandibular first molar. Root

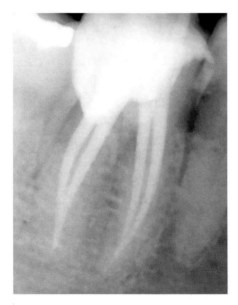

Figure 2.37

A mandibular first molar with four separate canals, two in each root.

- A working length radiograph should be taken at an angle to separate the mesial canals.
- The distal canal often exits on the side of the root face short of the anatomical apex, and therefore a file can appear short on a length estimation radiograph.

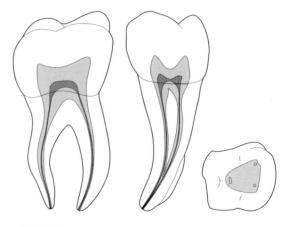

Figure 2.39

Mandibular second molar.

canal lengths are shorter, at 20 mm, and the average pulp volume is 32.9 mm^3. The C-shaped canal is more common in Mongoloid races; the mesial and distal canals become fused into a fin.

Clinical Points

- There may be only one mesial canal. The mesial and distal canals then lie in the mid-line of the tooth.
- The root canals are normally simpler than in the mandibular first molar.
- C-shaped canals can be extremely difficult to instrument and clean effectively. Ultrasonic irrigation is invaluable, in addition to allowing hypochlorite time to be effective.

Mandibular Third Molar

This tooth shows enormous variation; there may be one, two or three canals.

Clinical Point

- The mandibular third molar is usually more easily instrumented than the maxillary third molar, because the tooth tends to be tilted mesially, making access easier.

FURTHER READING

Black GV (1897). Descriptive anatomy of the human teeth, 4th edn. Philadelphia: SS White Dental Manufacturing Co.

Dummer PM, McGinn JH, Ress DG (1984). The position and topography of the apical constriction and apical foramen. *International Endodontic Journal* **17**: 192–198.

Fanibunda KB (1986). A method of measuring the volume of human dental pulp cavities. *International Endodontic Journal* **19**: 194–197.

Vertucci FJ (1984). Root canal anatomy of human permanent teeth. *Oral Surgery, Oral Medicine and Oral Pathology* **58**: 589–599.

3 PREPARATION PRIOR TO ENDODONTICS

CONTENTS • **Introduction** • **Caries** • **Pulpal Damage During Crown Preparation** • **Alternative Techniques for Tooth Substance Removal** • **Management of Deep Caries in a Vital Tooth** • **Management of Caries in the Non-vital Tooth** • **Teeth with Destruction of Marginal Ridges** • **Cracked Teeth and Fractures** • **Placing Orthodontic Bands** • **Crowned Teeth and Bridge Abutments** • **Temporary Crowns** • **Crown Lengthening** • **Orthodontic Extrusion** • **Further Reading**

INTRODUCTION

Before embarking on root canal treatment or retreatment, the practitioner should have an overall treatment plan and specific plans about restorations for teeth scheduled for root canal treatment. For example, if an existing crown needs to be replaced then root canal treatment may be made easier by removing it. In the case of a severely broken-down tooth, would an alternative to root canal treatment and subsequent crowning be more suitable (Fig. 3.1)? Other choices might be the addition of a tooth to a removable partial prosthesis, provision of a fixed bridge or an implant-retained prosthesis? Time spent on careful treatment planning will avoid unnecessary problems later.

Lack of coronal seal has now been highlighted as a significant cause of failure in root canal treatment. The quality of the coronal seal should be addressed from the start of treatment. Leaking restorations (Figs. 3.2, 3.3) and recurrent caries will allow the ingress of bacteria into the root canal system; the effectiveness of cleaning and shaping the root canal system will be compromised if there is a lack of good coronal seal. It is also important to achieve an effective seal with a rubber dam to prevent salivary contamination during root canal preparation.

Although the best view of the pulp floor is obtained when the tooth is broken down, the lack of sufficient tooth substance can make

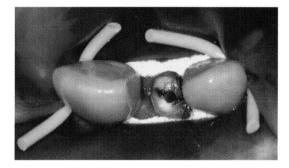

Figure 3.1

In this case a post-crown restoration on a maxillary lateral incisor has fractured. There is caries present and little tooth substance remaining. Would it be better to extract the tooth and replace it with an alternative restoration such as a bridge?

isolation difficult. Also, working length tends to be short, and it can be difficult to control this, as the rubber stop may move on the instrument. Severely broken-down teeth will normally benefit from some coronal build-up, such as the use of an orthodontic band to allow effective clamp placement and prevent salivary leakage during preparation or between visits. Complete restoration of the tooth, for instance with a permanent filling material before root treatment, is rarely necessary.

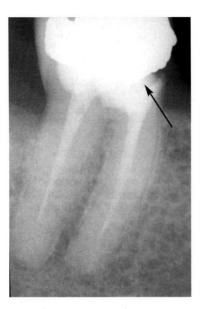

Figure 3.2

A radiograph showing a reasonable root canal treatment but poor coronal seal (arrowed).

CARIES

The dentist's primary aim in managing caries is to try and maintain the health of the dental pulp. However, in the case of deep carious lesions it can sometimes be difficult to ensure the appropriate removal of softened dentine whilst avoiding pulp exposure. Carious pulp exposure normally results in the mature tooth requiring root canal treatment. In this case all caries should be removed before root canal treatment is commenced.

The Dilemma of Deep Caries

There is now consensus amongst clinicians that during cavity preparation soft carious dentine at the amelodentinal junction and over the pulp should be removed. When preparing deep carious lesions in vital teeth clinicians find it difficult to know when to stop excavation. If pulp exposure can be avoided then root canal treatment may often be unnecessary in a tooth free of signs and symptoms. There is, however, no justification

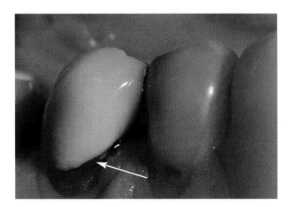

Figure 3.3

Leaking restorations do not provide a good coronal seal. The buccal margin of this full crown restoration has a marginal deficiency (arrowed) that could allow coronal leakage during root canal treatment if an access cavity were cut through the occlusal surface. It would be better in this case to remove the crown before root canal preparation and recement it temporarily between visits.

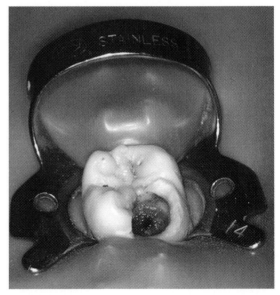

Figure 3.4

A molar tooth with active caries, which is lighter in colour.

for leaving carious dentine in the base of a cavity merely to avoid carrying out root canal treatment when there are signs or symptoms of pulpitis or pulp necrosis.

The colour of dentine can be used as an indicator of caries activity. Active caries tends to be light (Fig. 3.4). Hardness is a better indicator of disease activity, but requires subjective assessment, and is dependent on the sharpness of the probe and the pressure applied (Fig. 3.5). An alternative approach involves the use of an indicator dye; but there is some concern that this method may lead to unnecessary removal of the deepest layer of softened but not infected dentine.

There are many ways in which caries can be removed, from the routine to the experimental:

Mechanical rotary: Handpiece and burs
Mechanical non-rotary: Hand excavators, air abrasion, ultrasonics, sono-abrasion
Chemo-mechanical: Carisolv, Caridex
Photo-ablation: Lasers

Mechanical rotary techniques are the most widely used for caries removal. Carious dentine is most effectively removed using a round bur in a slow-speed handpiece with waterspray. Waterspray cools and lubricates the bur during cutting. The spray, by being directed at the cutting surface, prevents overheating and consequent pulpal damage; this has been shown experimentally. The larger the area of dentine that is being prepared the greater is risk of pulpal damage.

PULPAL DAMAGE DURING CROWN PREPARATION

The preparation of teeth for metal-ceramic crowns is potentially damaging to the pulp. Extensive amounts of dentine are removed, especially from the buccal surface, exposing many dentine tubules that can later be invaded by micro-organisms. Pulpal blood flow is also reduced owing to the action of adrenaline in local anaesthetic. The depth of a cavity, however, is of little significance until preparation extends to within 0.3 mm of the pulp tissue. Excessive drying of the cavity results in odontoblasts being aspirated into the dentine tubules; but this rarely results in permanent pulp damage.

ALTERNATIVE TECHNIQUES FOR TOOTH SUBSTANCE REMOVAL

There have recently been some new developments in techniques for caries removal. Chemo-mechanical techniques have shown good potential as a selective method of caries removal in lab-based experiments, and may be useful in deep carious lesions to prevent pulpal exposure. Air abrasion (Figs. 3.6, 3.7) using aluminium oxide particles will remove sound enamel and dentine very efficiently, but not carious dentine, as it is softer than the aluminium particles themselves. Alternative particles such as polycarbonate resin or alumina-hydroxyapatite are softer and may selectively remove carious dentine whilst sparing healthy tissue. Favourable results have also been reported for sono-abrasion of carious dentine with specialized diamond-coated tips.

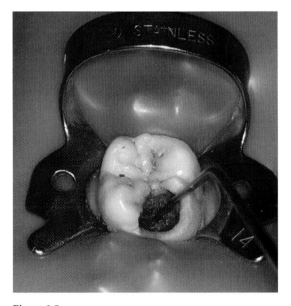

Figure 3.5

A probe can be used to test the hardness of caries.

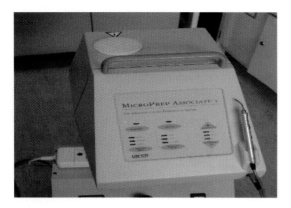

Figure 3.6

An air abrasion unit.

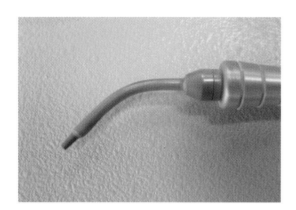

Figure 3.7

The air abrasion tip.

The pulp is remarkably resilient to irritation by micro-organisms. No focus of inflammatory cells is seen in the pulp until caries is within 1 mm, and only mild inflammation is seen microscopically when the advancing carious lesion is within 0.5 mm (Fig. 3.8). This is because the pulp dentine complex is able to protect itself from irritants by the mechanisms of tubular sclerosis and irritation dentine. When bacteria invade the irritation dentine severe inflammatory changes are seen in the pulp. Therefore if infected dentine is removed and the cavity is then sealed, the majority of pulps will survive. Bacterial leak-

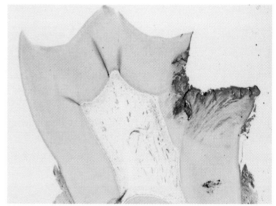

MANAGEMENT OF DEEP CARIES IN A VITAL TOOTH

Why?

To prevent irreversible damage to the pulp by bacterial microleakage, soft carious dentine is removed from the base of deep cavities. The tooth is then restored to function and the pulp protects itself by laying down irritation dentine. Leaving carious dentine may result in the bacteria causing pulp necrosis and further destruction of the tooth by the spread or recurrence of caries.

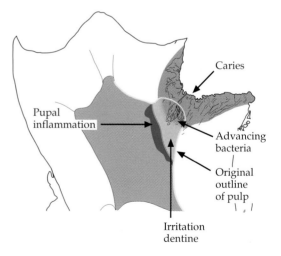

Figure 3.8

Histological section of advancing caries and corresponding diagram.

age occurs around most restorative materials after placement, and potentially can lead to pulpal inflammation. It is therefore imperative that measures are taken to seal the cavity following caries removal.

When?

Caries removal is carried out prior to the placement of a restoration. The pulp will protect itself from microleakage by tubular sclerosis (Fig. 3.9), formation of irritation dentine and inflammation; but measures need to be taken to prevent pulp damage before these biological processes have taken place. Lining the cavity for reasons of thermal protection or to prevent material irritation is unnecessary. Dentine has good insulation properties, and few restorative materials are irritant. Most of the original work on material irritancy has now been shown to be due to bacterial leakage and not to the materials themselves. Linings are therefore principally required to prevent bacterial leakage.

How?

All carious material is removed from the amelodentinal junction, and softened dentine is removed from the base of the cavity. The cavity can then be sealed using a variety of methods according to the overlying restorative material:
- Varnish
- Zinc oxide eugenol-based cement
- Composite and dentine-bonding agent
- Glass ionomer or resin-modified glass ionomer
- Poly acid-modified composite (compomer)

Varnish

Copalite varnish can be used to seal the prepared cavity; two coats are recommended to ensure complete coverage prior to placing amalgam. A varnish can also be used to seal exposed dentine following crown preparation.

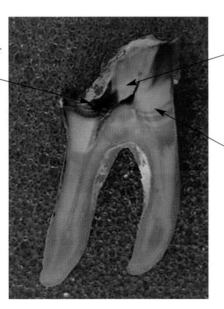

Microleakage under large amalgam restoration

Irritation dentine

Tubular sclerosis and dead tracts

Figure 3.9

The pulp will protect itself from microleakage by tubular sclerosis, formation of irritation dentine and inflammation.

Zinc Oxide and Eugenol-Based Cement

Eugenol-based materials prevent microleakage because they have an antibacterial action as eugenol is leached out. When treating deep carious lesions some operators suggest removing the bulk of the infected dentine and placing a fortified zinc oxide eugenol temporary filling for several months, as an indirect pulp cap (Fig. 3.10). The remaining small amount of carious dentine is removed at a later date, when it is hoped that the pulp will have laid down irritation dentine. The operator should beware, however, that the tooth is not necessarily healthy because it is symptom-free, as it may have become non-vital before placing the definitive restoration!

Composite Resin and Dentine-Bonding Agents

Modern composite resins placed following total etch procedures bond well to hydrated dentine, using primer and bond systems (Figs. 3.11–3.13). Calcium hydroxide liners are now rarely advocated to protect the dentine;

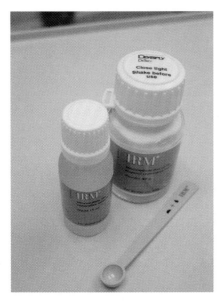

Figure 3.10

A reinforced zinc oxide eugenol cement such as IRM (Intermediate Restorative Material: Dentsply, Weybridge, Surrey, UK) is extremely useful in endodontics. The eugenol content is antibacterial.

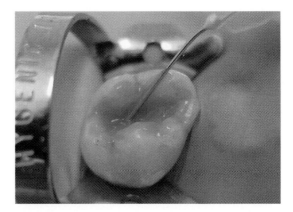

Figure 3.11

Etching dentine for composite bonding.

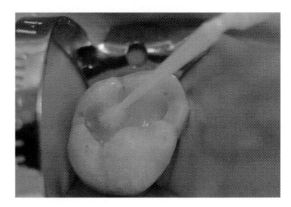

Figure 3.12

Addition of bonding agent to etched surfaces. These should not be over-dried.

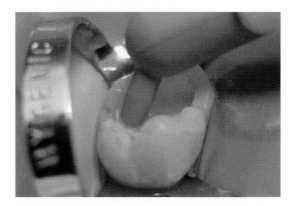

Figure 3.13

Composite is added in layers.

instead it is etched and protected with a bonding agent. Dentine-bonding agents provide a seal by penetrating dentine tubules and producing a hybrid layer. The materials are not irritant to pulp tissue. Poor technique and contamination with oil, saliva or blood may produce an inferior bond that allows microleakage leading to pulpal inflammation. It has been recommended that cavity margins are etched and sealed with a dentine-bonding agent following polishing of composite restorations to help prevent microleakage. Composites are now available in a range of viscosities, from flowable to packable. The flowable variety may be particularly useful to seal the cavity before placement of a higher-viscosity material.

Dentine-bonding agents used with bifunctional primers can be used to bond amalgam restorations, and may provide an element of seal.

Glass Ionomer

This material bonds to enamel and dentine, and can therefore be used to seal cavities prior to root canal treatment. The bond, as with most adhesive materials, is vulnerable to contamination. Glass ionomers undergo slow maturation that is affected by the degree of hydration. Glass ionomers can be particularly useful when placing an orthodontic band to protect endodontically treated teeth.

Resin-modified glass ionomers have significantly higher intermediate strength than conventional glass ionomers. They are ideally used in thick sections and are suitable for sandwich-style restorations with light-cured composite restorative materials. They can be used to seal cavities prior to root canal treatment.

Poly Acid-modified Composite (Compomer)

This material has properties similar to that of conventional composite, but uses slow water uptake from the oral environment to mediate the glass ionomer setting reaction. It can be used to build up a tooth prior to root canal treatment.

MANAGEMENT OF CARIES IN THE NON-VITAL TOOTH

Before a non-vital tooth is to be root treated the quality of coronal seal should be assessed. If the existing restoration has significant marginal deficiencies or there is evidence of recurrent caries, it should be removed. If a tooth is to be root canal retreated the operator should be questioning whether the demise of the previous root canal treatment could be due to coronal leakage around a poor restoration. It is now known that the quality of the coronal restoration as well as the quality of the root canal treatment affects the long-term outcome of root-filled teeth. Infected dentine is removed in exactly the same ways as with vital teeth. The quality of coronal seal is important during root canal treatment to prevent microleakage between visits and following root canal treatment. The cavities can be sealed with a reinforced zinc oxide eugenol material. Materials that bond to dentine and enamel can be useful where there is little tooth substance remaining, and may offer some protection from fracture during root canal treatment by preventing cusps from flexing.

TEETH WITH DESTRUCTION OF MARGINAL RIDGES

As restorations become more extensive, the inherent strength of the remaining tooth decreases.

Teeth with large MOD restorations and loss of the roof of the pulp chamber are vulnerable to fracture.

If there are any signs of cracks in a tooth that is to be root-treated, cusps have broken off, or the restoration is particularly large with vulnerable cusps remaining, it may be prudent to fit an orthodontic band before root canal treatment is started.

CRACKED TEETH AND FRACTURES

There is a difference between a cracked tooth (Fig. 3.14) and a longitudinally fractured tooth

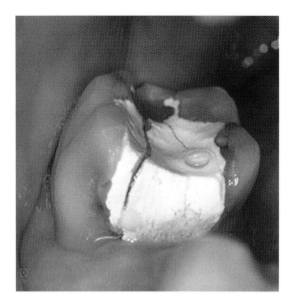

Figure 3.14

A cracked tooth with a crack running mesiodistally through the crown.

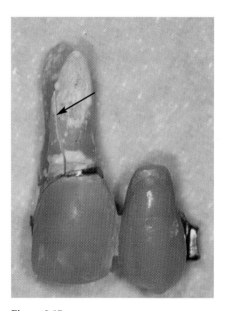

Figure 3.15

A fractured tooth with a longitudinal fracture (arrowed) in the root.

(Fig. 3.15). The latter involves movement of the two or more fragments, radiological signs, or bone loss associated with the root defect. Heroic attempts have been made to bond together longitudinally fractured teeth; however, the long-term prognosis is poor and extraction is usually the only treatment (Figs. 3.16–3.18).

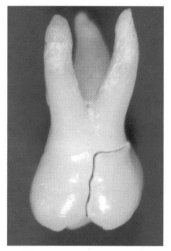

Figure 3.16

A cuspal fracture; the tooth can be restored with filling material.

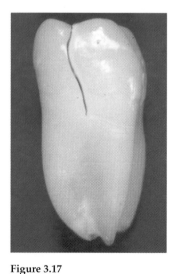

Figure 3.17

A severe cuspal fracture; root canal treatment and crown lengthening may be required. A subsequent crown will be required to prevent vertical root fracture.

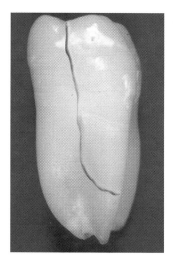

Figure 3.18

A longitudinal root fracture. This tooth would require extraction.

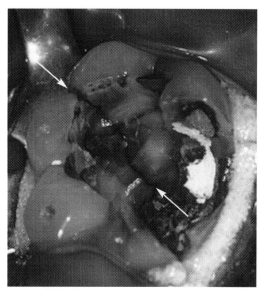

Figure 3.19

A crack (arrowed) running across the roof of the pulp in a buccal-lingual direction. The crack did not extend completely through the coronal tooth substance. As the tooth was non-vital it was root-treated and restored with a crown.

The treatment of cracked teeth, however, depends on the severity of the crack and the degree of inflammation within the pulp. Patients with a cracked cusp or tooth will often complain of pain on biting, especially when releasing from the bolus. This can be explained by the fact that the crack contains bacteria, which cause inflammation within the pulp. Chewing opens the crack, allowing oral fluids to flow in. As the tooth fragments snap back together fluid movement is produced in the dentine tubules, eliciting pain in the inflamed pulp. If the tooth were vital and showed no signs of irreversible pulpitis then treatment would involve removal of the fractured cusp and placement of a new restoration. A pinned amalgam restoration may be suitable. Alternatively, the tooth could be restored with a cusp coverage restoration to reduce the stress applied to the cusps during mastication.

A crack may run across the roof of the pulp chamber (Fig. 3.19). If the tooth is vital and symptom-free then a sealing restoration, such as zinc oxide and eugenol cement, glass ionomer cement or a dentine-bonded composite may prevent bacterial ingress sufficiently for root canal treatment to be avoided. The tooth must be protected from stresses that could result in propagation of the crack, and a full coverage restoration may be required. Cracks that run across the pulp chamber floor may have become infected with bacteria and are therefore more difficult for the clinician to manage. Some teeth will not be savable, while in others it may be possible to seal the pulp floor and place a cusp coverage restoration, prolonging the life of the tooth for several years.

Teeth requiring endodontic treatment may benefit from the placement of a band to prevent fracture. Following root canal treatment it is normally recommended to place a full coverage crown or cusp coverage restoration to protect the tooth from subsequent fracture.

PLACING ORTHODONTIC BANDS

Why?

Unfortunately, a number of posterior teeth undergoing root canal treatment are lost as a

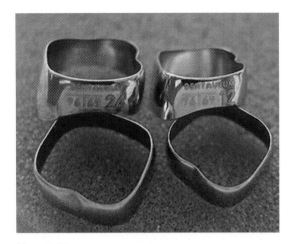

Figure 3.20

A collection of orthodontic bands.

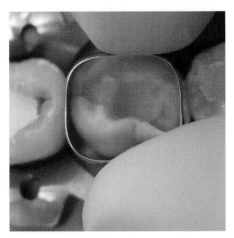

Figure 3.22

Checking the fit of a band.

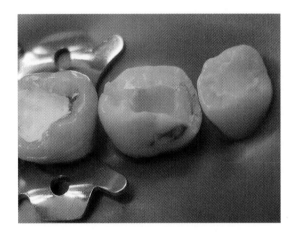

Figure 3.21

A fractured first molar tooth that requires placement of an orthodontic band prior to root canal treatment.

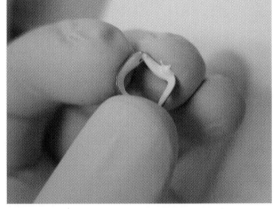

Figure 3.23

Zinc phosphate cement is placed on the band prior to seating. Excess cement is carefully removed.

result of fracture. If a band is fitted to the tooth before endodontic treatment, this will help prevent propagation of a crack or fracture. It will also help improve rubber dam isolation of a severely broken-down tooth.

When?

If a posterior tooth shows early signs of fracture, such as crack-lines in the enamel, or is significantly broken down, so that isolation with rubber dam is difficult, a band can be fitted. Teeth with subgingival cavity margins may benefit from the placement of a band to achieve a good coronal seal for root canal treatment. Occasionally, the tooth might be crown-lengthened before root canal treatment.

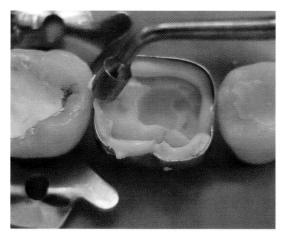

Figure 3.24

Seating the band using an amalgam plugger.

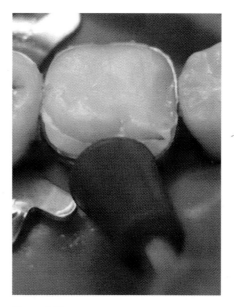

Figure 3.26

The margins are polished with an abrasive rubber cup.

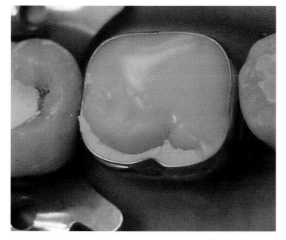

Figure 3.25

The cavity in the banded tooth is filled with glass ionomer.

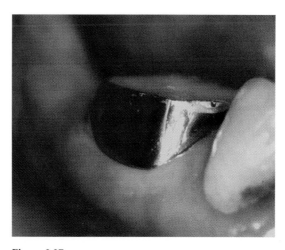

Figure 3.27

A well-fitting orthodontic band in place on a mandibular first molar.

How?

Orthodontic bands are made of stainless steel and can be purchased without brackets (Fig. 3.20). They are manufactured to fit maxillary and mandibular premolars and molars. A band is selected that fits snugly around the tooth (Figs. 3.21, 3.22). The occlusion on the band may need to be adjusted. Bands are bonded using zinc phosphate or glass ionomer cement

(Fig. 3.23). It may be necessary to ease the band into position using an amalgam plugger or a tooth slooth (Fig. 3.24). If the tooth is severely broken down then the entire band can be filled with glass ionomer (Fig. 3.25). This will allow the tooth to be isolated using rubber dam, and also gives a good coronal seal between visits during endodontic treatment. The edges are polished with an abrasive rubber cup (Fig. 3.26). Once bonded the occlusion is rechecked with articulating paper, and any high spots are removed with a diamond bur (Fig. 3.27).

It is often advisable to leave rubber dam placement to the following visit, when the luting cement will have set completely.

Copper Bands

Copper bands have long been used in dentistry, for example as a matrix for amalgam core fabrication and for taking impressions. They can be used in a similar manner to orthodontic bands to protect teeth that are vulnerable to fracture or to build up teeth that are severely broken down. These bands are also cemented with zinc phosphate or glass ionomer cement. They tend to be cheaper than orthodontic bands, but require more customization and are less well tolerated by patients (they can taste metallic).

Metal Shell Crowns

Metal shell crowns can be used as temporary restorations. These are filled with either glass ionomer or zinc oxide eugenol cement. The margins often need to be adjusted, smoothed and polished. Ideally the margins should be supra-gingival to prevent damage to the periodontal ligament and plaque accumulation (Fig. 3.28).

CROWNED TEETH AND BRIDGE ABUTMENTS

Crowned Teeth

The dilemma when root-treating a crowned tooth is whether to remove the restoration or not. Placing a rubber dam clamp on a tooth that has been prepared for a crown can be difficult. If the margins of a cast restoration are poor or appear to be leaking then the restoration is probably best removed. It can always be replaced as a temporary measure using glass ionomer or zinc oxide eugenol cement after caries removal. This will act as a sound

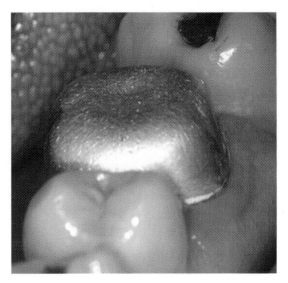

Figure 3.28

A simple metal shell crown filled with zinc oxide and eugenol cement has been used to seal an endodontically treated tooth prior to permanent restoration. The margins are supragingival and smooth, ensuring good periodontal health.

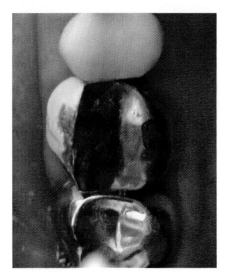

Figure 3.29

The crown on the first molar has gross caries under the distal margin that will compromise coronal seal during root canal treatment.

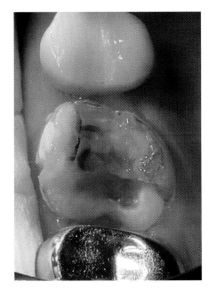

Figure 3.30

The crown was partially split and then elevated and the caries removed.

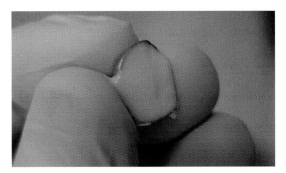

Figure 3.31

The crown is cleaned and filled with glass ionomer.

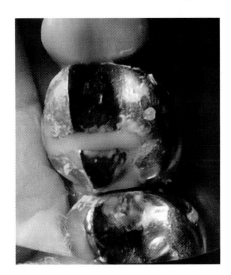

Figure 3.32

The crown is replaced.

temporary restoration and aid rubber dam isolation (Figs. 3.29–3.33).

It may not be possible to locate the pulp space and remove all the carious dentine working through an access cavity in a crown.

Removing Crowns

Why?
A crown may be removed:

• To make access easier
• To aid removal of caries
• To improve the coronal seal
• To improve visualization of cracks.

When?
If a crown is due to be replaced then it may be easier to remove it prior to endodontic treatment. However, if the crown is sound, root canal treatment may be carried out through an access cavity in the occlusal surface. This cavity can be restored following root canal treatment.

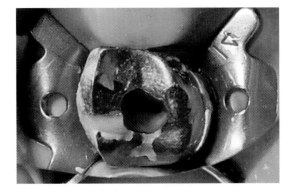

Figure 3.33

Rubber dam can be fitted more easily and an access cavity cut through the crown.

How?

Crowns can be removed using:

- *Ultrasonics*
  There are special tips produced for Piezon ultrasonic handpieces (EMS, Forestgate, Dallas, TX, USA) to vibrate cast restorations (Figs. 3.34, 3.35). A groove may need to be cut in the restoration into which the tip can be placed. The unit is run on maximum power with waterspray. An ultrasonic scaler tip can also be used, but will probably be slightly less effective. Scaler tips are useful for breaking up cement around the margins of poorly fitting crowns. The restoration is then elevated by carefully rotating a chisel.

- *Chisel or flat plastic*
  A chisel or flat plastic inserted into a marginal deficiency can be sufficient to break the cement bond. Care must be taken not to place too great a force on the crown so that the core or tooth substance is fractured. Forces should always be applied along the long axis of the plane of insertion of the restoration (Figs. 3.36, 3.37).

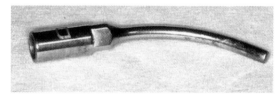

Figure 3.34

An ultrasonic tip for vibrating posts and crowns.

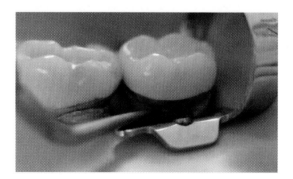

Figure 3.35

A CT4 tip being used to remove a crown.

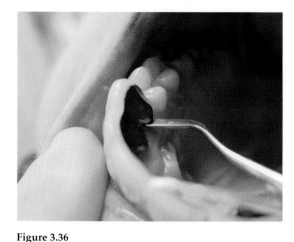

Figure 3.36

A flat plastic inserted under the margin of a crown to remove it.

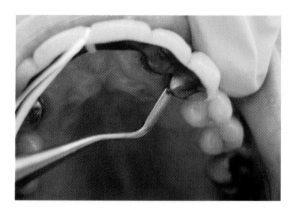

Figure 3.37

To avoid fracture, the flat plastic must not apply lateral forces.

- *Crown tapper*
  The crown tapper consists of a weight on a rod with various hooks for inserting under the crown margin. The hook is held firmly in place and the weight gently tapped on the stop at the end of the rod. Force is applied along the path of insertion of the crown. The momentum of the weight may be sufficient to break the cement lute (Figs. 3.38, 3.39).

- *Pneumatic crown remover*
  This handpiece fits on to the dental airline and allows controlled pneumatic forces to

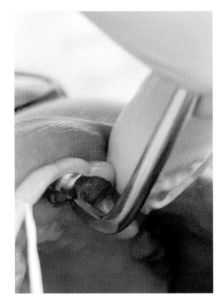

Figure 3.38

The tip of the crown tapper is inserted under the margin.

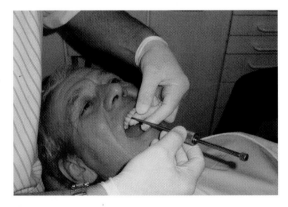

Figure 3.39

The crown tapper being used to remove a bridge.

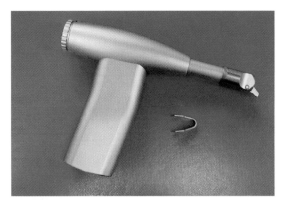

Figure 3.40

The Kavo pneumatic crown and bridge remover.

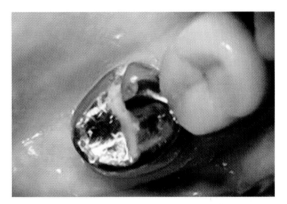

Figure 3.41

This crown has been sectioned prior to removal.

be applied to the crown via a specially designed pair of forceps (Fig. 3.40).

• *Sectioning*
  A crown can be partially sectioned by cutting a groove from the gingival on to the occlusal surface (Fig 3.41). A chisel is then placed in the groove and twisted, allowing the crown to be flexed and thereby break-

ing the cement. If the crown is resistant to removal then it can be sectioned completely and the pieces elevated.

Bridge Abutments

It is useful to check if a bridge abutment has decemented and become loose by placing a probe under the pontic and applying pressure coronally (Fig. 3.42). If the restoration is loose then the bridge abutment will move. Air bubbles in the saliva may be seen at the margin of the bridge–tooth interface. If the abutment has decemented then it is prudent to remove the restoration. If the abutment has

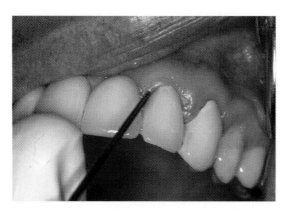

Figure 3.42

Placing a probe under a bridge to check retention.

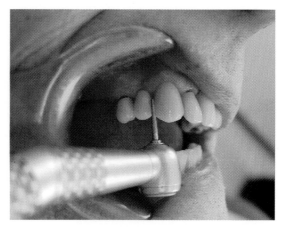

Figure 3.43

Sectioning a bridge. The maxillary right second premolar is the post-retained distal abutment for a three-unit bridge. The tooth requires root canal retreatment. The entire bridge could be removed in order to gain access. Alternatively, the bridge could be sectioned. In this case, the bridge was cut through mesial to the maxillary first premolar.

been loose for some time then the coronal tooth tissue will often be grossly carious.

Alternatively, a bridge can be sectioned into smaller pieces. The abutment and pontic can be removed. Care should be taken if the remaining bridge section is left as a cantilever, because excessive occlusal forces could lead to the demise of the remaining abutment.

Removing a Bridge

Bridges can be removed using the same techniques as those for removing crowns. It can be useful to attach a length of dental floss to the bridge before removal in case it is accidentally dislodged into the back of the patient's mouth.

When a bridge has multiple retainers it may be necessary to cut grooves in the separate retainers, allowing the lute to be broken on each before attempting removal.

Sectioning a Bridge

Metal ceramic bridges can be sectioned through appropriate approximal contacts using a long tapered diamond bur on the ceramic and a cross-cut tungsten carbide bur on the metal (Fig. 3.43). It is useful to attach a length of dental floss to the portion that is to be removed in case it is dislodged into the patient's mouth, especially if the abutment has debonded. The cut surface of the remain-

ing section of the bridge that is to remain in place should be polished with a rubber wheel. If the remaining section becomes cantilevered then the occlusion must be examined, as excessive force placed on the remaining bridge components could lead to fracture of the remaining abutment. In such a case it may be better to leave the abutment as a single unit.

TEMPORARY CROWNS

Temporary crowns are constructed:

- To restore the occlusion and prevent over-eruption and tilting
- To prevent bacterial penetration by coronal leakage
- To prevent damage to the prepared tooth
- To prevent damage to the periodontium and food packing
- To restore the aesthetic appearance of the teeth.

Temporary crown forms are available for anterior teeth constructed from polycarbonate and acrylic (Fig. 3.44). These are usually filled with methacrylate resin (e.g. Trim: Dentsply) and seated on the tooth by the practitioner. Preformed crowns require careful adjustment to achieve a good fit and an aesthetic result. They should be cemented with a suitable cement to prevent microleakage (Fig. 3.45).

It is probably easier to construct well-fitting temporaries from a preoperative alginate impression. If the tooth is broken down then the alginate impression can be modified using an excavator or scalpel. Custom-cast temporaries made from bis-acryl resin (e.g. Protemp: ESPE, Seefeld, Oberlay, Germany or Luxatemp: DMG, Hamburg, Germany) have a good appearance and are quick to make, and the margins are easy to trim. The temporary can be adjusted with a medium grit sandpaper disc or a stone (Fig. 3.46).

Even if a posterior tooth has been root-filled it is important to place a well-fitting temporary, for the above reasons. If the filled root canals are left exposed to the oral environment then they could become re-infected.

Metal shell crown forms can be used (as discussed earlier). They are filled with zinc oxide eugenol cement and seated into place.

Modern syringe-mixed resins (Protemp, Luxatemp) make the fabrication of custom-cast temporary restorations much easier. These are cast using a preoperative alginate impression. The temporary crowns should be cemented with a eugenol-based temporary cement. Leakage is more of a problem with long-term temporary restorations, and if they

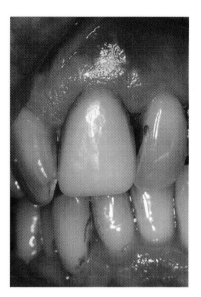

Figure 3.45

A preformed acrylic temporary used to restore the tooth during endodontic treatment. As there was limited coronal tooth substance remaining the temporary acrylic crown was completely filled with glass ionomer cement and bonded in place. This provided a good seal during root canal treatment and avoided the need for a temporary post crown.

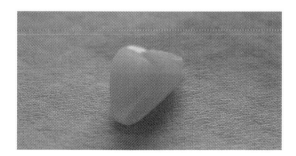

Figure 3.44

A preformed acrylic crown; it is useful to roughen the internal surface before bonding.

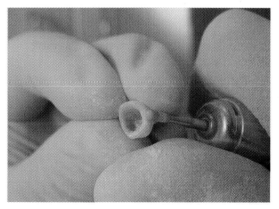

Figure 3.46

Trimming a custom-cast temporary restoration before cementation.

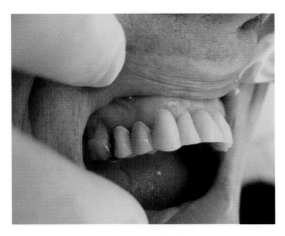

Figure 3.47

Long-term provisional restorations for a complex restorative case.

become loose, patients should be instructed to have them recemented immediately (Fig. 3.47).

CROWN LENGTHENING

Why?

Periodontal surgery can be used to:

- Increase the clinical crown to give adequate retention for crowns; this may be necessary for a root-filled tooth that is severely broken down. Carrying out crown lengthening prior to endodontic treatment allows easier isolation with rubber dam and provisional restoration.
- Subgingival restoration margins and recurrent caries can be exposed. It should then be easier to ensure good coronal seal of such a restoration.
- Exploration of superficial cracks. Cracks that are supragingival can usually be sealed with a restorative material. A deep vertical crack that extends down the root surface may so reduce the prognosis of the tooth that extraction becomes the treatment of choice.

When?

In some cases where there has been attrition and/or erosion of teeth the available crown height may be insufficient for satisfactory retention. The retention form of the crown preparation can be improved greatly with the use of seating grooves (Fig. 3.48).

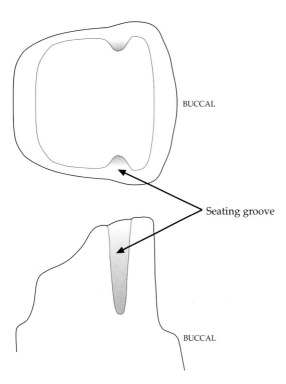

Figure 3.48

The retention form of the crown preparation can be improved greatly with the use of seating grooves.

ORTHODONTIC EXTRUSION

When?

Orthodontic extrusion can sometimes be used to reposition a tooth that has a subgingival horizontal root fracture communicating with the gingival sulcus. Orthodontic extrusion is usually complicated, and requires the services of an orthodontist. There can be difficulty providing a suitable provisional restoration, and in the long term it must be possible to restore the tooth, otherwise orthodontic extrusion is not indicated.

The practitioner must consider whether a suitable alternative to trying to save a badly fractured tooth would be more successful.

FURTHER READING

Banerjee A, Watson TF, Kidd EAM (2000). Dentine caries excavation: a review of current clinical techniques. *British Dental Journal* **188:** 476–482.

Feiglin B (1986). Problems with the endodontic–orthodontic management of fractured teeth. *International Endodontic Journal* **19:** 57–63.

Kirkevang L-L, Ørstavik D, Hörsted-Bindslev P, Wenzel A (2000). Periapical status and quality of root fillings and coronal restorations in a Danish population. *International Endodontic Journal* **33:** 509–511.

Saunders WP, Saunders EM (1994). Coronal leakage as a cause of failure in root canal therapy: a review. *Endodontics and Dental Traumatology* **10:** 105–108.

4 ISOLATION

CONTENTS • **Isolation** • **Rubber Dam Frames** • **Rubber Dam Clamps** • **Rubber Dam Punch** • **Rubber Dam Forceps** • **Lubricants, Tape and Wedgets** • **Sealants** • **Rubber Dam Placement** • **Rubber Dam Kit** • **Quick Single Tooth Isolation Method** • **Multiple Teeth Isolation** • **The Split-dam Technique** • **Using Wingless Clamps** • **Practical Solutions to Isolation Problems**

ISOLATION

The use of rubber dam is essential for good-quality endodontic treatment. With experience it can be placed quickly and efficiently, and it improves treatment for both operator and patient (Fig. 4.1).

When?

Any tooth that is undergoing an endodontic procedure should be isolated with rubber dam. This includes a range of procedures, from an endodontic emergency such as pulp extirpation and placement of medicaments to more complex and time-consuming root canal retreatment.

Why?

There are many benefits from the use of rubber dam:

- To prevent the accidental aspiration or swallowing of instruments, irrigants, fragments of tooth and restorative materials. Practitioners who do not use rubber dam could be considered negligent and place themselves at risk of litigation should an accident occur.
- To prevent contamination of the access cavity and root canal system with saliva.

- To reduce and control the aerosol of microbes and saliva produced when using a turbine handpiece. In addition, the patient does not have a mouth full of water.
- The soft tissues are retracted, affording them protection while the patient is being treated. The inquisitive tongue is kept out of the tooth being treated.
- Rubber dam allows unimpeded vision of the tooth that is being treated. This is especially useful when using a surgical microscope.
- The operative field can be dried, and mirror fogging caused by breathing is prevented.
- Rubber dam produces a watertight seal that allows the safe use of sodium hypochlorite and other disinfectants as irrigants.
- Treatment is quicker and more pleasant for both the patient and the clinician.

How?

Rubber Dam

Rubber dam is usually made of latex, and comes in sheets of varying thickness. The sheets range from thin to extra-heavy, depending on thickness, and are 150 mm square. There are many different colours, flavours and aromas! (Fig. 4.2). For patients who have an allergy to latex, a silicone (non-latex) rubber dam is available (Fig. 4.3).

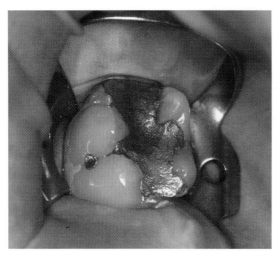

Figure 4.1

Well-placed rubber dam aids endodontic treatment.

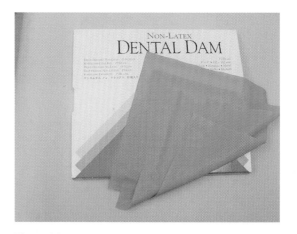

Figure 4.3

Non-latex dam is made of silicone.

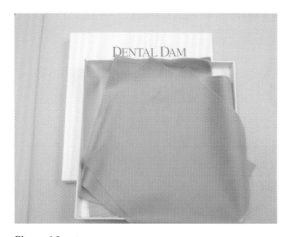

Figure 4.2

Different colours, sizes and grades of rubber dam are available.

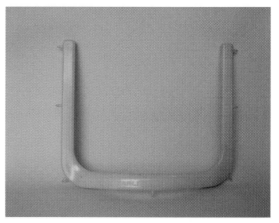

Figure 4.4

Plastic 'U' shaped frame.

RUBBER DAM FRAMES

Modern frames are constructed from plastic so that they can remain in place during radiography. There are two basic types, Young's frame, which has a 'U' shape (Fig. 4.4) and the Nygard–Ostby (Fig. 4.5), which is oval in shape. Frames were originally constructed from metal (Fig. 4.6), and were radiopaque, so that they needed to be removed to avoid obscuring important detail on radiographs.

RUBBER DAM CLAMPS

Most rubber dam clamps are now manufactured from stainless steel, as this resists corrosion much better than plated steel. They come with or without wings. Clamps are essential

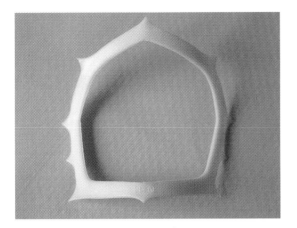

Figure 4.5

Nygard–Ostby frame.

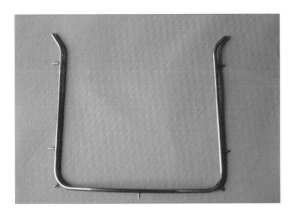

Figure 4.6

Metal frames are no longer used.

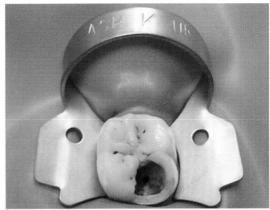

Figure 4.7

K clamp (Dentsply, Weybridge, Surrey, UK).

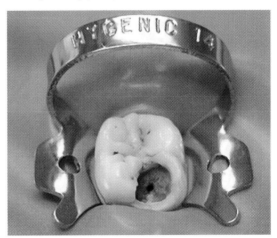

Figure 4.8

14 clamp (Hygenic, Akron, OH, USA).

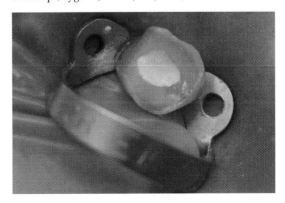

Figure 4.9

EW clamp (Dentsply).

for retaining rubber dam on posterior teeth, and very valuable for anterior teeth. Fully erupted teeth can be isolated with an appropriate clamp, although partially erupted teeth and broken-down teeth can be difficult to isolate. Manufacturers have produced a large range of clamps. These can be identified by catalogue number or letter, depending on the make (Figs. 4.7–4.11).

The advantage of a winged clamp on a molar tooth is that both clamp and dam can be placed on the tooth simultaneously, thereby speeding up the process. When a wingless clamp is used on a molar tooth, it is

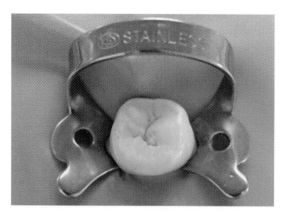

Figure 4.10

1 clamp.

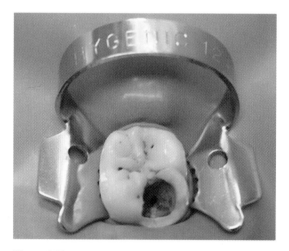

Figure 4.11

13A clamp (Hygenic).

normal to place the clamp first, and place the dam over it. Most anterior teeth can be isolated with a small winged clamp; but if stability is a problem, a wingless clamp is almost always successful. For endodontic treatment it is usually only necessary to isolate and clamp the tooth being treated. In a small number of instances additional teeth may need to be isolated. Broken-down posterior teeth may be difficult to clamp properly; sometimes a more retentive wingless clamp may be successful, or alternatively an ortho-

dontic band may be cemented around the tooth to allow easier clamping with a winged clamp.

RUBBER DAM PUNCH

There are many different types of rubber dam punch; some punch a single hole (Fig. 4.12) while others have a mandrel that allows the operator to select one of several holes of different diameters, ranging from 0.5 to 2.5 mm (Figs. 4.13, 4.14). The punch and mandrel must be aligned to cut a clean hole so that the rubber dam does not tear when stretched. For endodontic applications the single hole punch is entirely satisfactory.

RUBBER DAM FORCEPS (Fig. 4.15)

Forceps are used to place, align and remove rubber dam clamps. The shape of the tips is critical for easy clamp placement. The tips should have a smaller diameter than the holes in the clamp, to allow removal of the forceps

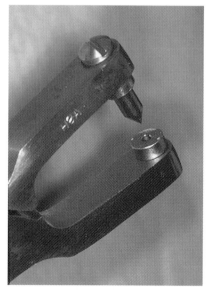

Figure 4.12

The mandrel of a single hole punch.

Table 4.1 *Rubber dam clamps placed in groups according to catalogue letter and equivalent number*

Clamp	Description of lettered clamp
K (3, 4, 5, 7A, 8, 10, 11, 8U(67), 26, 26A, 7, 8A)	The authors have found this clamp to be an extremely versatile molar clamp, suitable for most situations.
EW (0, 00, 2, 2A, 9, 15, 18A)	A universal clamp for all incisors, canines and premolars, where only limited gingival retraction is required.
A (14, 18A)	Very retentive universal molar clamp. Especially useful where the tooth is not fully erupted or is broken down.
AW (4, 5, 8, 14, 8AUW, 145)	Very retentive universal molar clamp (including deciduous second molars). Especially useful where the tooth is not fully erupted.
BW (3, 4, 5, 6, 7A, 8, 10, 11, 8U(67), 26, 26A, 8A, 27A)	Bland clamp for all well-erupted molars.
C (6, 9, 15, 9UW, 212)	For gingival retraction buccally around incisors, canines and premolars.
DW (27)	For small molars and first deciduous molars and some premolars.
E (0, 00, 2, 2A, 9, 15, 18A)	Universal winged clamp for all incisors, canines and premolars, where only limited gingival retraction is required.
FW (14A)	Molar clamp, useful when the molar is not fully erupted.
G (1, 2, 2A)	This clamp is designed to fit third molars, and is also useful for incisors, canines, and premolars.
GW (1, 2, 2A)	A useful clamp for incisors, canines, premolars and upper third molars.
HW (14W, 14LH, 14AD)	The arch of this clamp has been set further back to enhance access to the tooth, e.g. for manipulating matrix bands or taking impressions.
JW (26A)	For large molars, with minimal tooth substance.
L (0)	Universal clamp for all incisors, canines and premolars, where only limited gingival retraction is required.
M (2)	Clamp for molars and premolars.
NW (4UW, W4)	A medium-sized wingless molar clamp, fairly retentive.
PW (5UW, W5)	Wingless retentive molar clamp.

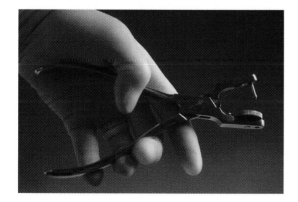

Figure 4.13

A multihole punch.

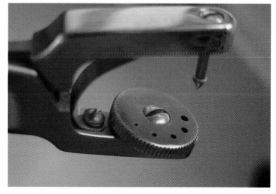

Figure 4.14

The mandrel of a multihole punch.

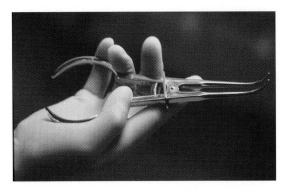

Figure 4.15

Rubber dam forceps.

following clamp placement. Sometimes it is necessary to reduce the size of the tips of newly manufactured forceps; this can be done with a diamond bur or a carborundum disc (Fig. 4.16).

LUBRICANTS, TAPE AND WEDGETS

Silicone lubricant or shaving foam can be used to ease the placement of rubber dam through tight interproximal contacts, although they are not often required for endodontic applications. Dental tape can be used to take rubber dam through a contact point and can then act as a retainer.

Wedgets (Hygenic: Fig. 4.17) or strips of rubber dam (Fig. 4.18) can be used to retain the dam instead of a clamp in the front of the mouth. This is especially useful in the anterior region when it is necessary to use a split-dam technique.

SEALANTS

Various caulking agents have been marketed to help seal around rubber dam. Oraseal putty (Ultradent, South Jordan, UT, USA; Fig. 4.19) and caulking are examples. For larger deficiencies or in the absence of a commercial caulking agent Cavit (ESPE, Seefeld, Oberlay, Germany) or Kalzinol (Dentsply) are useful.

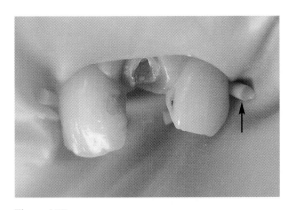

Figure 4.17

Wedgets (arrowed) used to secure a split dam.

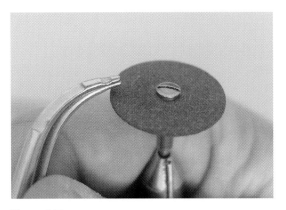

Figure 4.16

Adjusting rubber dam forceps with a carborundum disc.

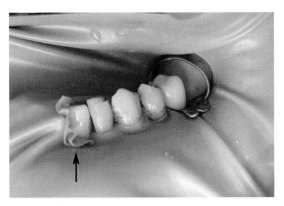

Figure 4.18

A strip of rubber (arrowed) used to secure the mesial end of a multi-tooth isolation.

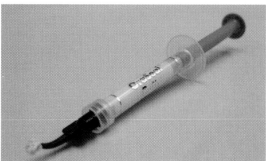

Figure 4.19

Oraseal putty.

On occasions, some elastomeric impression material can be used.

RUBBER DAM PLACEMENT

Fitting rubber dam to a frame (Figs. 4.20–4.27).

RUBBER DAM KIT

The rubber dam can be pre-assembled and laid out before use. This speeds up placement (Fig. 4.28).

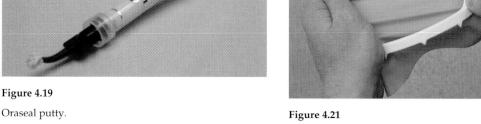

Figure 4.21

The sheet is secured along one side of the frame with light tension.

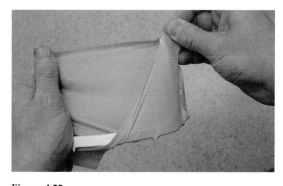

Figure 4.22

The bottom of the rubber dam sheet is then looped over the end of the frame, thereby fixing this side.

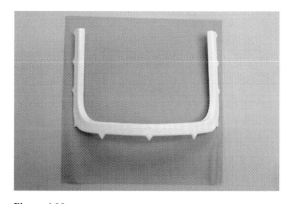

Figure 4.20

A 'U' style frame and rubber dam sheet.

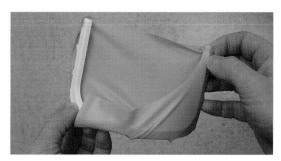

Figure 4.23

The process is repeated on the opposite side.

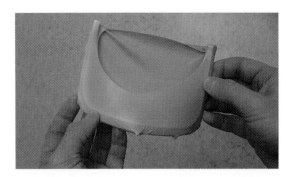

Figure 4.24

When both sides have been folded a deep gutter is created.

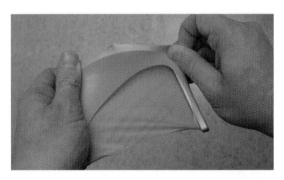

Figure 4.25

Pushing the overhanging dam back over the corners of the frame, on one side.

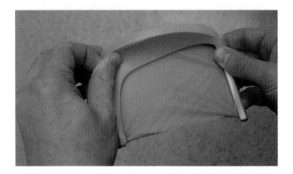

Figure 4.26

Then the other.

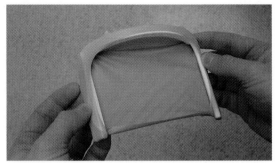

Figure 4.27

The dam is ready for placement.

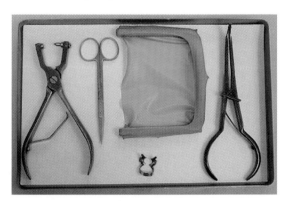

Figure 4.28

A rubber dam kit.

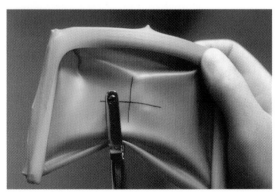

Figure 4.29

A cross is imagined on the frame and a hole punched in the relevant quadrant. The punch is positioned over the mandibular left quadrant in this picture.

QUICK SINGLE TOOTH ISOLATION METHOD

1. The rubber dam is fitted on to the rubber dam frame so that a gutter is created (see Figs. 4.20–4.27).
2. Imagine a cross in the centre of the rubber dam; a hole is punched in the relevant quadrant (Fig. 4.29).
3. A winged clamp is selected and placed in the rubber dam (Figs. 4.30, 4.31).
4. Using forceps the clamp is introduced on to the tooth. The operator must be careful to make sure that the soft tissues are not trapped (Fig. 4.32).
5. The clamp is allowed to close on to the tooth in the correct position, and the rubber dam is then released from the clamp wings using a flat plastic or fingers (Figs. 4.33–4.36).
6. Sealant can be applied for extra protection if necessary (Fig. 4.37).

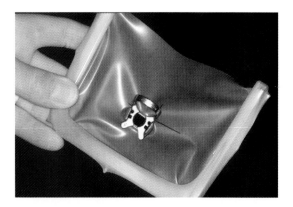

Figure 4.31

The clamp is fitted to the rubber dam to isolate a mandibular right molar.

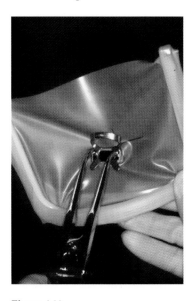

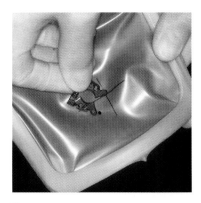

Figure 4.30

A winged clamp is selected. In this case a hole has been punched to isolate a mandibular right molar.

Figure 4.32

Using forceps the dam assembly is introduced to the tooth.

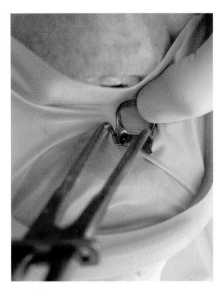

Figure 4.33

Isolation of a mandibular left molar. The forceps are used to carry the dam, frame and clamp to the tooth.

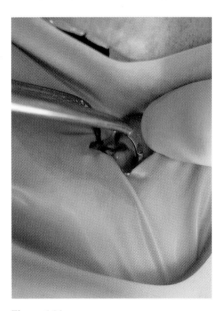

Figure 4.34

The clamp is introduced over the tooth and guided with the clinician's finger.

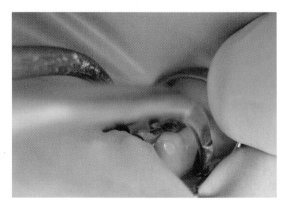

Figure 4.35

Once the clamp is fully seated the forceps are removed.

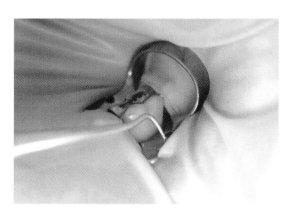

Figure 4.36

The dam is released from the wings.

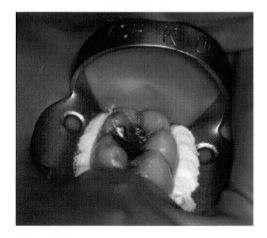

Figure 4.37

In this case, sealant has been applied for extra protection.

MULTIPLE TEETH ISOLATION

(This is much more time-consuming than single tooth isolation, and so is only used when it is required for endodontics.)

1. Multiple holes are punched for the relevant teeth. The positions can be marked on the dam using a ball-point pen (Fig. 4.38).
2. A clamp is selected for the most posterior tooth in the arch.
3. The rubber dam is again fitted with the frame and clamp.
4. Using forceps, the clamp is positioned and successive teeth are isolated by stretching and forcing the dam between the interproximal contacts. A second clamp or strip of rubber can be used to retain the dam anteriorly (Figs. 4.39, 4.40).
5. Placing rubber dam through tight interproximal contacts can be difficult. Stretching the dam will make it thinner, and makes 'knifing' (Fig. 4.41) it through a tight contact easier. Waxed dental floss can also be used to ease dam through a difficult contact. It can then be tied off to help retain the rubber.

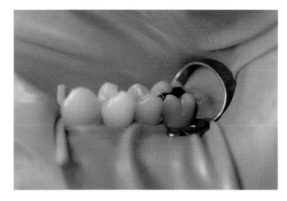

Figure 4.39

A clamp has been placed on the most posterior tooth and the dam fitted over the teeth to be isolated.

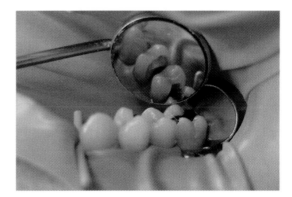

Figure 4.40

The mesial aspect of the dam has been retained with a wedget. The edges of the dam are inverted into the gingival sulcus and provide a good seal.

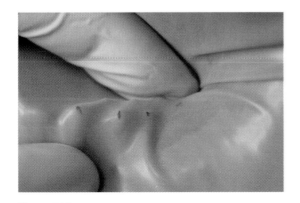

Figure 4.38

Marking holes for multiple isolation.

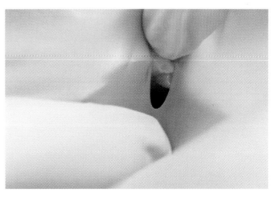

Figure 4.41

Knifing dam through a tight contact.

THE SPLIT-DAM TECHNIQUE

This technique is especially useful when attempting to isolate a badly broken-down tooth, perhaps where there are subgingival margins and the standard method has failed. It may also be useful when attempting to isolate abutment teeth on a bridge, those that have been prepared for crown restorations or teeth that are not fully erupted.

1. Two holes are punched in the rubber dam that correspond to the teeth either side of that which is being isolated (Fig. 4.42).
2. A slit is cut in the dam to join the two holes (Fig. 4.43). The rubber dam can be retained with clamps, wedgets, or strips cut from the corners of a rubber dam sheet. Sometimes with anterior teeth extra retention is not required (Fig. 4.44).
3. The split gives poor isolation; therefore a caulking agent is required to seal the defective margins (Fig. 4.45).

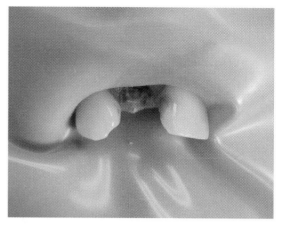

Figure 4.44

A split dam has been fitted quickly and easily. It will prevent anything from dropping into the back of the patient's mouth. An EW clamp could also have been used in such a situation.

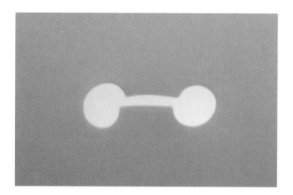

Figure 4.42

Two holes punched in the rubber dam for a split-dam technique.

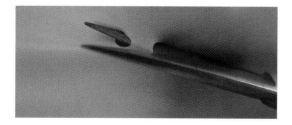

Figure 4.43

A slit is cut between the holes.

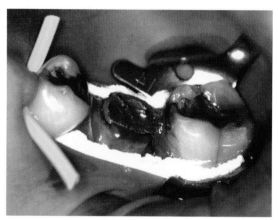

Figure 4.45

Caulking used to seal a split dam in the posterior region. The molar tooth had been prepared for a crown, and clamp placement was difficult.

USING WINGLESS CLAMPS

The wingless clamp (Fig. 4.46) is tried on the tooth that needs to be isolated to check for stability and fit. A length of dental floss should be tied to the clamp, as this aids retrieval should it be dropped in the patient's mouth during application. Dental floss can be passed through a hole in the clamp, wound

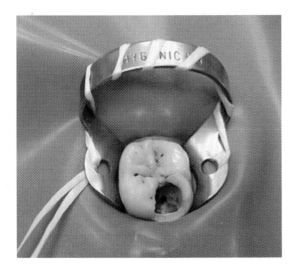

Figure 4.46

A wingless clamp used in the posterior region. Floss has been tied to the bow during placement.

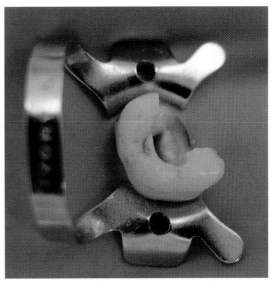

Figure 4.47

A poorly fitting clamp will not retain the dam satisfactorily. On the palatal aspect of this tooth the clamp does not fit properly, the dam has slipped and there is a gap through which leakage will occur.

around the bow and tied off in the opposite hole. The rubber dam is punched and stretched over the clamp; it is easier to pass the dam over the bow of the clamp first and then over each side.

PRACTICAL SOLUTIONS TO ISOLATION PROBLEMS

The rubber dam splits:

1. Check that the rubber dam punch is cutting a clean hole in the dam: a complete circle should be removed following punching.
2. Check that the mandrel is meeting the anvil at the correct angle to cut evenly.
3. Make a larger hole in a new sheet of dam by punching two overlapping holes; the dam is stretched less and should not tear.

The rubber dam clamp comes off the tooth:

1. Check that the clamp is the correct size for the tooth (Fig. 4.47).
2. Clamps need to be flexed a few times when first purchased before use, and can become distorted after regular use.

3. When isolating a posterior tooth make sure that there is some slack in the rubber dam from side to side on the frame to reduce the tension across it when it is on the tooth.

Bridges

1. If the entire bridge is to be isolated, then a split-dam technique can be used (Fig. 4.48).
2. Single abutments can be isolated with a single isolation technique; small gaps near the pontic can be filled with caulking (Fig. 4.49).

Badly Broken-Down Teeth

1. Use a split-dam technique, and seal the edges with a caulking agent.
2. Use a subgingival clamping technique, but

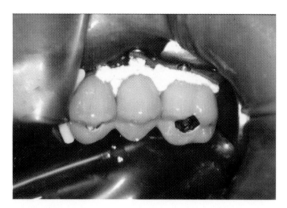

Figure 4.48

Isolation of a bridge using a split-dam technique.

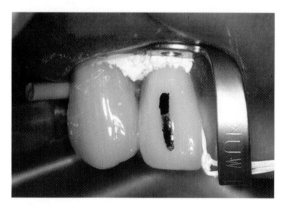

Figure 4.49

An EW clamp has been used in the isolation of these double-abutted bridge retainers. Gaps around the dam and pontic have been filled with caulking. A line has been drawn on the buccal surface of the crown to give an indication of the root angulation during access preparation.

try to avoid traumatizing the gingivae.

3. Build the tooth up with glass ionomer or zinc phosphate cement and an orthodontic band. Dentine pins may occasionally be required, but should be placed sparingly. Use of a band is particularly useful if the tooth is a lone standing posterior tooth, and will also improve the coronal seal between appointments (Fig. 4.50).

Situations where the crown length is longer than the height of the clamp arch, preventing proper seating:

1. Clamp the tooth more coronally.
2. Use wedgets or strips of rubber dam in a non-clamp technique.
3. Use orthodontic separators to secure the rubber dam around the neck of the tooth. A heavier grade of dam may also help.
4. If the teeth are to be used for over-dentures, then reduce the clinical height before placement of the rubber dam.

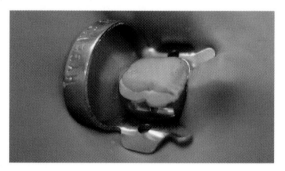

Figure 4.50

A clamp can easily be fitted to a tooth once it has been restored with an orthodontic band.

5 ROOT CANAL PREPARATION

CONTENTS • **Rationale** • **Access Cavity Preparation** • **Hand Instruments** • **Preparation Techniques** • **Hand Preparation** • **Mechanical Preparation Techniques** • **Further Reading**

RATIONALE

Microbiology

Apical periodontitis is caused by microbial infection of the root canal system. Successful treatment is dependent on the control of this microbial infection. An understanding of the microbiology of apical periodontitis is a prerequisite for effective treatment.

The General Microbial Flora

With the development of anaerobic culturing techniques and sampling methods an insight into the microbial flora of infected root canals has become possible. Nowadays there are sophisticated techniques for identification of bacteria that do not rely on culturing methods. Indeed some bacteria that can be identified by genetic techniques are non-cultivable. Apical periodontitis is typically a polymicrobial infection dominated by obligately anaerobic bacteria. Normally only a few species are isolated from any one case. *Porphyromonas endodontalis* is a species that seems to predominate in infected root canals. Others include: *Streptococcus, Enterococcus, Actinomyces, Lactobacillus, Peptostreptococcus, Eubacterium, Propionibacterium, Prevotella, Fusobacterium, Eikenella, Capnocytophaga* and *Wolinella.*

There are positive and negative interactions between bacterial species as they compete in the ecological niche of the root canal. Environmental conditions such as the amount of oxygen, availability of nutrients and host defence mechanisms will affect colonization. Bacteria infect the main canals and lateral canals; they also may infect dentine by spreading down dentinal tubules. The periradicular tissues are normally separated from the flora in the root canal by a dense wall of polymorphonuclear leukocytes, and it is rare to see bacteria in the periapical tissues unless there is acute apical periodontitis.

Rationale for Root Canal Preparation

Because the root canal system of a tooth is often extremely complex it is difficult to disinfect it completely and quickly. It may be that the best attempts of the operator merely reduce the residual bacterial load to a non-pathogenic number, or change the resident flora sufficiently to allow periapical healing, but this has not been proved. These microbes and their by-products can be removed by a combination of mechanical and chemical means.

Mechanical removal relies on the ability of the operator to remove infected pulp and dentine from the surfaces of the root canal by planing the walls; infected material in the lumen of the root canal will be removed. In nearly all cases this is impossible to achieve, partly because the instruments cannot actually contact all the internal surfaces and also because attempting to remove *all* the infected dentine would severely weaken the tooth. That is why chemically active irrigants are used to destroy colonies of micro-organisms. Instrumentation of the root canal is carried out to produce a pathway for the delivery of an antibacterial irrigant to all the ramifications of the root canal system. It also makes space for medicaments and the final root canal filling.

Bacterial colonies may form themselves into multilayered biofilms, which can be difficult to remove, as they adhere to the canal wall, while other microbes congregate in suspension. Irrigants must be delivered in sufficient volume and concentration to be effective against these colonies. Sodium hypochlorite irrigant is inactivated by its action on organic material, and must be replenished.

ACCESS CAVITY PREPARATION

Preoperative Radiograph

A preoperative radiograph should normally be taken using a paralleling device, as this produces an image that is almost actual size. The radiograph must show the entire tooth and at least 2 mm of bone surrounding the root apices (Fig. 5.1). Images of root canals can become superimposed on radiographs and sometimes it will be necessary to take more than one view from different angles to interpret the complex arrangement of multi-rooted teeth.

The preoperative radiograph(s) will allow an assessment of basic anatomy: number of roots, size of pulp chamber, fit of coronal restoration, caries, pulp stones, curvature of root canals, likelihood of lateral canals, iatrogenic damage (perforations and fractured instruments). When a tooth has been

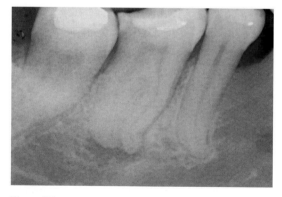

Figure 5.1

A good-quality radiograph of the mandibular first molar which requires root canal treatment.

crowned it is very important to assess the position of the pulp space in relation to the artificial crown, or else the access cavity may be misdirected.

Why? Aims of Access Cavity Preparation

The access cavity should be designed to allow debridement of the pulp chamber and enable root canal instruments to be introduced into the canals without bending—i.e. for straight-line access. The tooth must be caries-free and any restorations with deficient margins must be removed.

All necrotic pulp remnants must be removed from the pulp chamber, to prevent infected pulp material being pushed further into the canals and causing recontamination between visits. Necrotic material and breakdown products may also be responsible for staining dentine.

There should be some degree of resistance form to the completed access cavity; this ensures that temporary restorations are not dislodged between visits and a coronal seal is achieved.

How? Location of Access Cavity

Historically access cavity designs have been standardized according to the type of tooth. Although the final cavity shape may resemble the standardized form, using modern techniques the underlying pulp chamber should dictate the final shape. Small modifications to the shape may be needed to allow straight-line access to all the root canals.

The Lid-off Approach to Access Cavity Preparation (Fig. 5.2)

1. Estimate length
2. Penetrate to the pulp chamber
3. Lift off the roof with a bur in a pulling action
4. Refine the access cavity.

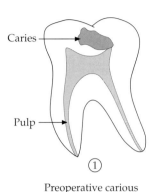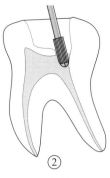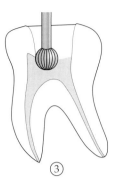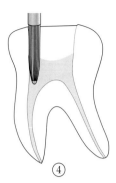

Caries

Pulp

① Preoperative carious exposure

② Dome-ended fissure bur is used to penetrate pulp chamber

③ Roof of pulp chamber removed with round bur

④ Non end-cutting bur is used to 'lift lid' of pulp chamber and refine cavity

Figure 5.2

Access cavity preparation: 'lid-off technique'.

Estimating the Depth

The depth of the roof of the pulp chamber can be estimated from the preoperative radiograph (Fig. 5.3).

Access is first made to this depth using a tungsten carbide or diamond bur, FG557 or FG541, in a turbine (Fig. 5.4). Pre-measuring will help prevent perforation of the pulp floor during access cavity preparation. The bur is directed towards the axis of the largest canal in multi-rooted teeth, for example the palatal root of maxillary molars and the distal root of mandibular molars. Locating this canal first makes orientation easier and subsequent identification of other canals more predictable. Further dentine can be removed with a long-shank low-speed round bur in a pulling action (Fig. 5.5). The remainder of the roof of the pulp chamber can now be removed using a non end-cutting bur, FG332 safe-ended diamond or FG safe-ended TC Endo-Z (Maillefer, Ballaigues, Switzerland: see Fig. 5.4). The non-cutting end can be safely guided over the floor of the pulp chamber whilst removing dentine from the walls of the cavity.

To gain straight-line entry into some canal orifices it may be necessary to enlarge the access in specific areas: for example to gain access to the curved mesiobuccal canal of the maxillary first molar tooth (Fig. 5.6).

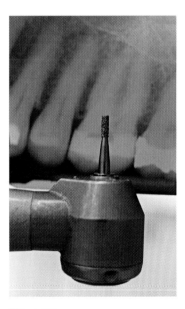

Figure 5.3

The depth of the pulp chamber can be estimated from a preoperative radiograph.

The orifices of the root canals can now be located. Some teeth have a variable number of root canals, and the clinician should be aware of how many canals are likely to be found in each tooth (Figs. 5.7–5.12, Table 5.1).

Table 5.1 *Number of roots and canals likely to be encountered in various types of tooth*

Tooth	Roots	Canals	Comments
Maxillary central incisor	1	1	The orifice normally lies apical to the incisal edge. The canal shape is wider buccolingually.
Maxillary lateral incisor	1	1	The orifice normally lies apical to the incisal edge. The canal shape is wider buccolingually.
Maxillary canine	1	1	The canal is wider buccolingually in the coronal aspect but becomes rounder in the apical region.
Maxillary first premolar	2	1 (35%) 2	Canal orifices lie buccally and palatally and the separate canals may be superimposed on the radiograph.
Maxillary second premolar	1	1 2 (50%)	Generally a single orifice and single canal.
Maxillary first molar	3	3 4 (>60%)	Mesial canal orifices may lie under a lip of dentine.
Maxillary second molar	3	3 (55%) 4	Similar to first molar.
Maxillary third molar	1–3	1–3	Variable anatomy.
Mandibular incisors	1	1 2 (40%)	Usually a single orifice, but the canal may bifurcate and converge in the apical third. As canals are located buccally and lingually, they may be superimposed on a radiograph.
Mandibular canine	1	1 2 (14%)	Resembles maxillary canine.
Mandibular first premolar	1	1 2 (2–5%) 3	Usually a single orifice. Lingual branches off the main canal (buccal) may produce 2 or 3 canals.
Mandibular second premolar	1	1	Chamber wider buccolingually.
Mandibular first molar	2 3	3–4 4	Usually two roots and three canals. Mesial orifices are located buccal and lingual to the midline. In 45% of mesial roots the two canals converge in a wide fin. A single supernumerary distolingual root can be present. The distal root has two canals in 38% and the two orifices lie equidistant to the midline. Occasionally the distal canal has one orifice and the canal bifurcates.
Mandibular second molar	2	3 C-shaped	C-shaped canals most common in Mongoloid races.
Mandibular third molar	1–3	1–3	Variable anatomy.

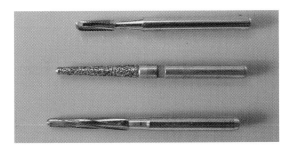

Figure 5.4

Burs for preparing an access cavity. The Jet Beaver dome-ended fissure bur (top: Beavers Dental, Morrisburg, Ontario, Canada) will cut through most restorations. Safe-ended diamond or Endo-Z burs are used to refine the preparation.

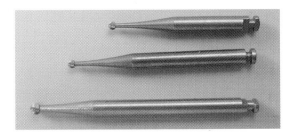

Figure 5.5

Round burs with different shank lengths (top: standard length bur). Medium- and long-shanked burs are useful in endodontics.

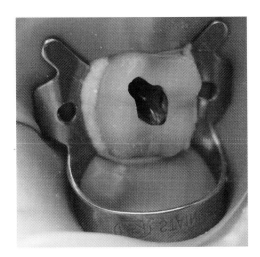

Figure 5.6

The access cavity has been modified in order to gain straight-line access to the mesiobuccal canal of this maxillary molar.

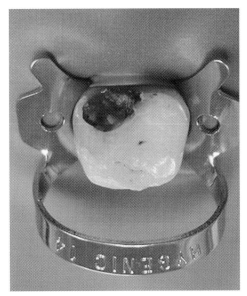

Figure 5.7

A carious maxillary molar with pulpal exposure.

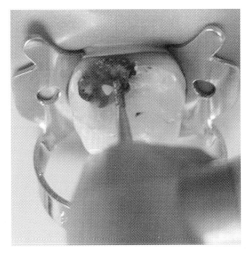

Figure 5.8

The cavity outline is prepared with a diamond bur (541).

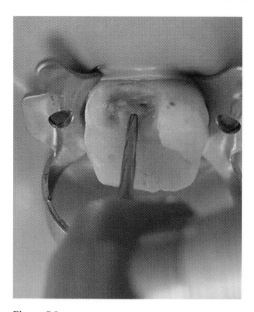

Figure 5.9

An Endo-Z non end-cutting tungsten carbide bur is inserted into the pulp chamber to remove the 'lid' of the pulp chamber.

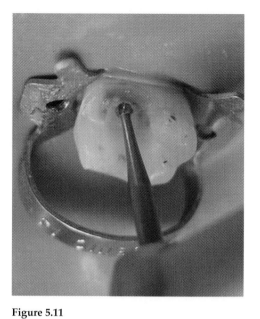

Figure 5.11

Remaining carious dentine is removed using a round bur.

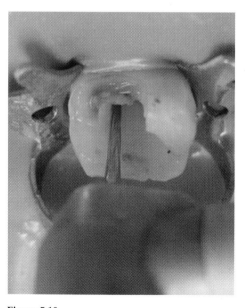

Figure 5.10

The access is refined with the Endo-Z bur.

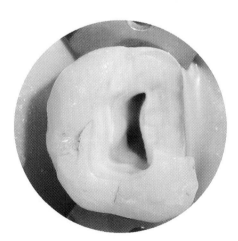

Figure 5.12

The completed access cavity gives straight-line access to all the canals.

The Pulp Floor Map

The floor of the pulp chamber can be read like a map. The dentine on the base of the chamber is generally darker (Figs. 5.13, 5.14) than that of the walls, and will normally indicate the lateral extent of the pulp chamber. This junction can be used to explore the extent of the pulp chamber.

An endodontic probe (e.g. DG16, Hu Friedy, Chicago, IL, USA) is a double-ended long probe designed for the exploration of the pulp floor and location of root canal orifices. A long-shanked excavator may also be helpful for removing small calcifications and obstructions when locating canals (Fig. 5.15).

Troubleshooting Access Cavity Preparation

Calcifications

Pulp stones and irritation dentine formed in response to caries and/or restorations may make the location of root canal orifices difficult. Special tips for ultrasonic handpieces (Fig. 5.16) are invaluable in this situation, as they allow the precise removal of dentine from the pulp floor with minimal risk of perforation. In the absence of a special tip a pointed ultrasonic scaler tip can be used to remove pulp stones from the pulp chamber.

Ultrasonic tips are best used with irrigant. Occasionally they may be used without, and a Stropko irrigator (Obtura Corporation, Fenton, MO, USA: Fig. 5.17) is then useful for

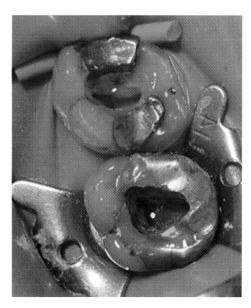

Figure 5.14

The access cavities in these maxillary molars have been prepared conservatively but give good straight-line access to the root canals.

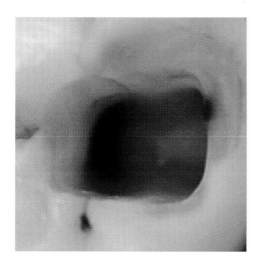

Figure 5.13

The pulp floor is generally darker than the walls of the cavity.

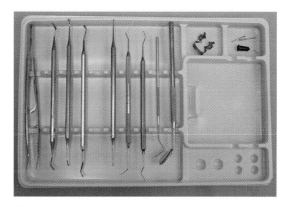

Figure 5.15

A typical preparation tray of instruments for endodontic treatment (left to right): college tweezers, flat plastic, ball-ended burnisher, amalgam plugger, excavator, DG16 probe, Briault probe, periodontal probe, mirror, number 14 clamp, Jet dome-ended fissure bur, Endo-Z bur, fine bore tip for Stropko irrigator.

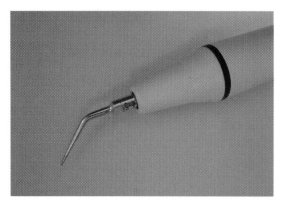

Figure 5.16

An ultrasonic tip for removal of dentine on the pulp floor.

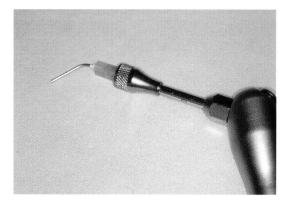

Figure 5.17

The Stropko irrigator.

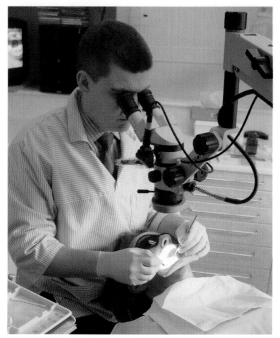

Figure 5.18

An operating microscope.

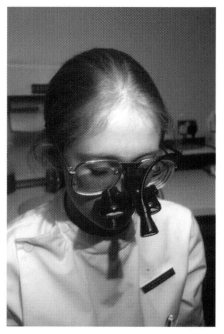

puffing away dentine chips. A solution of 17% EDTA is excellent for clearing away the area under exploration, as it removes the smear layer. Flood the pulp chamber with EDTA solution and allow it to stand for 1–2 minutes. Dentine chips and other debris can then be washed away with a syringe of sodium hypochlorite.

Sclerosed Canals

Illumination and magnification are vital for the location of sclerosed root canals. The endodontist would use a surgical microscope (Fig. 5.18), while a general dental practitioner might have loupes (Fig. 5.19) and a headlight available. A thorough knowledge of the

Figure 5.19

Loupes give excellent magnification and illumination.

anatomy of the pulp floor and the likely location of the canal orifices is essential. Chelating agents such as EDTA are of little use in the location of sclerosed root canals, as the chelating agent softens the dentine indiscriminately and may lead to the iatrogenic formation of false canals and possibly perforation. If the pulp chamber is filled with irrigant, bubbles can occasionally be seen appearing from the canal orifice. Occasionally dyes, such as iodine in potassium iodide or methylene blue, have been used to demonstrate the location of canal orifices.

Canal orifices tend to be located at an imaginary point directly apical to the original location of the cusp tip.

Dentine needs to be removed very carefully when attempting to locate sclerosed canals. Ultrasonic tips such as the CT4 design are very useful for precise removal of dentine from the floor of the pulp chamber. Long-shanked low-speed size 2 (ISO 010) round burs can be used with care.

If the canal is completely sclerosed for several millimetres apical to the pulp floor then instruments should be advanced gradually, removing small increments of dentine. It may be necessary to take radiographs to check that the ultrasonic tip or drill is in the correct position in relation to the root canal to avoid perforation of the root. The operator can easily become disorientated.

Unusual Anatomy

Good radiographic technique should alert the practitioner to unusual anatomy, such as C-shaped canals. The C-shaped canal may have the appearance of a fused root with very fine canals (Fig. 5.20). If confronted with a pulp chamber that looks unusual the dentine areas on the pulp floor map should give some idea of the location of root canals, and of the relationship of the floor to surrounding tooth structure.

Angulation of the Crown

If the extracoronal restoration of the tooth is not at the same angle as the long axis of the root, or a tooth is severely tilted, then great care must be taken to make the access cavity preparation in the long axis of the tooth to

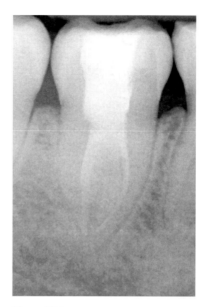

Figure 5.20

A radiograph of a 'C'-shaped canal in a mandibular second molar.

avoid perforation. In teeth with particularly long crowns it can also be difficult to locate the root canal. It may be appropriate in some rare instances to make initial penetration of the pulp chamber without the rubber dam in situ. This allows correct angulation of the bur, as the operator is not distracted by the angulation of the crown. As soon as the access cavity is fully prepared the rubber dam should be applied. It is important to make sure that the rubber dam clamp is positioned squarely on the tooth and perpendicular to the long axis of the root, as it will give a guide for access cavity preparation. This is very important in incisor teeth, where an incorrectly placed clamp can lead to perforation.

Restorations

Unless there are obvious signs of marginal deficiencies or caries then full crown restorations can generally be retained, with the access cavity being cut through the restoration. Diamond burs are very effective for cutting through porcelain restorations, while a fine cross-cut tungsten carbide bur, e.g. the Jet

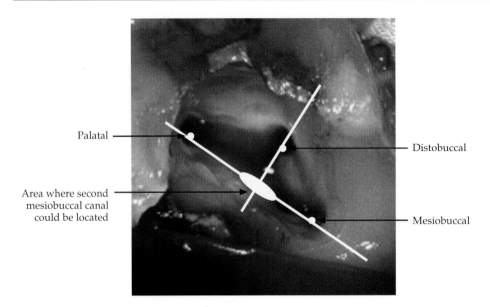

Figure 5.21

Location of the second mesiobuccal canal in the maxillary first molar.

Beaver bur, is particularly useful for cutting through metal.

Posts

Posts should be identified from the preoperative radiograph. When cutting the access cavity maximum post material should be retained to make its later removal easier. Core material may need to be removed from around a post to facilitate subsequent removal of the post.

The Location of 'Extra' Canals

The second mesiobuccal canal of maxillary molars (Fig. 5.21): There is a second mesiobuccal canal in approximately 60% of maxillary molars; it often lies under a lip of dentine on the mesial wall of the access cavity (Figs. 5.22, 5.23). Location of the orifice can be made by visualizing a point at the intersection between a line running from the mesiobuccal to the palatal canal and a perpendicular from the distobuccal canal. The lip of dentine in this area can be removed using an ultrasonic CT4

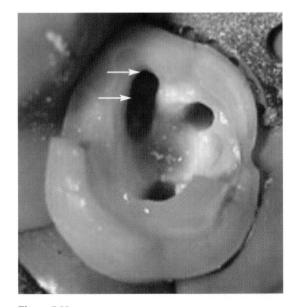

Figure 5.22

A lip of dentine has been removed using a round bur to uncover the two mesiobuccal canals (arrowed) in this maxillary molar.

tip or a size 2 round bur. There is often an isthmus between the main mesiobuccal canal and the second mesiobuccal (Fig. 5.24); this can be traced until the orifice is located. The pulp floor map should be followed to avoid overzealous exploration in the incorrect direction.

Four canals in mandibular molars (Fig. 5.25): Four canals are found in approximately 38% of mandibular molars. If the distal canal does not lie in the midline of the tooth, then a second distal canal should be suspected. The canals are often equidistant from the midline.

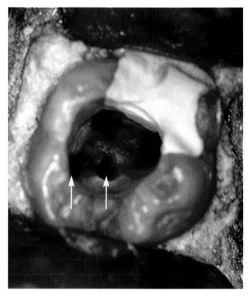

Figure 5.23

The location of the two mesiobuccal canals (arrowed) can clearly be seen in this maxillary molar following preparation.

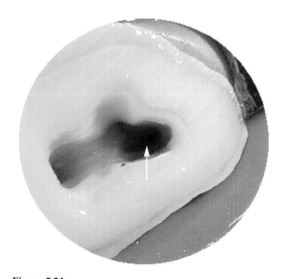

Figure 5.24

In this case the lip of dentine has been removed using ultrasonics to reveal an isthmus (arrowed).

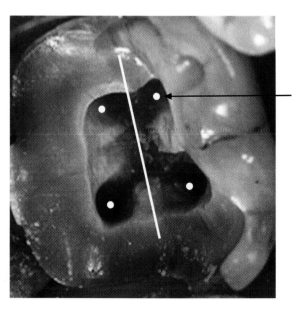

Distal canal orifices lie equidistant to midline

Figure 5.25

Location of a second distal canal in the mandibular first molar.

Careful exploration with a CT4 ultrasonic tip or round bur should uncover the orifice. It may be necessary to take a radiograph from a different angle to confirm the presence of the second distal canal.

Two canals in mandibular incisors (Fig. 5.26): The incidence of two canals in lower incisors may be as high as 41%. A common reason for failure of root canal treatment in these teeth occurs when a second canal has not been located and is consequently not cleaned. Canals may be missed owing to incorrect positioning of the access cavity. If access is prepared too far lingually then it may be impossible to locate a lingual canal. To gain entry into a lingual canal the access cavity may sometimes need to be extended very near to the incisal edge.

Two canals in a mandibular premolar (Fig. 5.27): The highest reported incidence of two canals in mandibular premolars is 11%. There are rarely two orifices. The lingual canal normally projects from the wall of the main buccal canal at an acute angle. It can usually be located by running a fine (ISO 08 or 10) file with a sharp bend in the tip along the lingual wall of the canal.

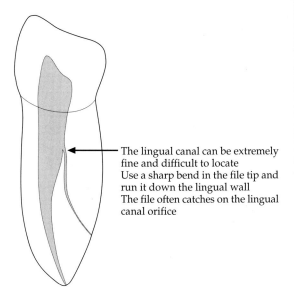

The lingual canal can be extremely fine and difficult to locate
Use a sharp bend in the file tip and run it down the lingual wall
The file often catches on the lingual canal orifice

Figure 5.27

Location of the lingual canal in mandibular premolars.

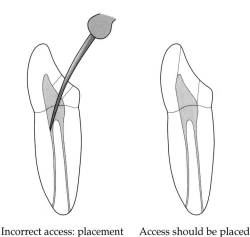

Incorrect access: placement too far lingually prevents entry into lingual canal

Access should be placed more incisally; straight-line entry into buccal and lingual canals can then be achieved

Figure 5.26

Location of the lingual canal in mandibular incisors.

HAND INSTRUMENTS

Endodontic research has shown how different instruments and materials behave within the confined space of the root canal system during instrumentation. In parallel with advances in hand instruments come new preparation techniques. These developments can occur so rapidly, however, that the chicken often precedes the egg!

Instrumentation techniques where apical preparation is carried out at the start of treatment have been superseded by crown-down techniques, in which the coronal element of the root canal is prepared first. The actions with which files can be used have been analysed, and now many modern methods of instrumentation use a balanced force motion as opposed to filing. With the introduction of highly flexible materials such as nickel–titanium alloys it has been possible to produce instruments with tapers that are greater than the original stainless steel hand files, without losing flexibility; such instruments are invaluable for tapering the root canal preparation predictably.

As new instrument systems are produced,

new preparation techniques evolve. The morphology of the root canal space is highly variable, however, and one preparation technique cannot be applied to every situation. It is perhaps more useful to develop and understand basic concepts of root canal preparation. These can then be implemented to master the diversity of root canal systems with which the dentist may be faced. This approach also allows the clinician to modify his or her current technique as new instruments are produced. Unfortunately no one system can be a panacea. An understanding of endodontic concepts and a consequent adaptation of techniques with which the clinician is conversant will avoid the unfortunate accumulation of expensive equipment that becomes redundant when it fails to deliver its promises! There are no secrets to effective root canal preparation: just practice, patience and persistence.

Hand Files and Reamers

For the last forty years root canal instruments have been produced to international standards. There are specifications for dimensions, fracture resistance, stiffness and colour coding of endodontic files and reamers. Reamers have fewer turns per unit length than the equivalent-sized file.

Material

Endodontic files and reamers are mainly manufactured from stainless steel, although carbon steel, titanium and nickel–titanium are also used. The different materials give the instruments different properties, which in turn affect the way in which they should be used.

Tip Design

The tip of the instrument can have various shapes. Originally instrument tips were sharp and had a cutting action; but non-cutting (bullet-shaped) tips are now available that allow the instrument to slide along the outer curvature of a root canal, allowing prepara-

tion to be centred on the original canal curvature.

There is a non-linear increase in the diameter of tip sizes between consecutive instruments. To address this, one manufacturer produced intermediate sizes between 10 and 30. Golden Mediums (Maillefer) are available in ISO sizes 12, 17, 22 and 27. Another method of reducing the uneven 'jumps' in diameter between sizes has been to produce instruments with a uniform increase in diameter between consecutively sized instruments. Series 29 (Dentsply, Weybridge, Surrey, UK) instruments have a 29% increase in tip size between instruments.

Restoring Force

This is the force produced by a file when it resists bending. The restoring force for a nickel–titanium instrument is 3–4 times less than that for an equivalent-sized stainless steel file. The restoring force increases with

Table 5.2 *ISO size and colour coding*

Colour	Size	Tip (mm)*
Pink	06	0.06
Grey	08	0.08
Purple	10	0.10
White	15	0.15
Yellow	20	0.20
Red	25	0.25
Blue	30	0.30
Green	35	0.35
Black	40	0.40
White	45	0.45
Yellow	50	0.50
Red	55	0.55
Blue	60	0.60
Green	70	0.70
Black	80	0.80
White	90	0.90
Yellow	100	1.00
Red	110	1.10
Blue	120	1.20
Green	130	1.30
Black	140	1.40

*Nominal size at tip if it were not modified to be, for example, safe-ended.

file diameter: i.e. files get stiffer as their diameter increases.

Taper

The standards for instruments specify that hand files have a 0.02 taper; i.e. the diameter of the instrument increases by 0.02 mm per mm along the length of the instrument. However because nickel–titanium is superelastic, it has been possible to create flexible instruments with larger tapers such as 0.04, 0.06, 0.08, 0.10 and 0.12.

Instrument Design

Endodontic files can be twisted from square, rhomboid or triangular stainless steel blanks, or machined. The standardized length of a file or reamer blade is 16 mm. Reamers normally have fewer flutes/blades per unit length than an equivalent file, and are intended for use in a rotary action. Nickel–titanium instruments need to be machined using computer-assisted manufacturing (CAM), as the material is superelastic and cannot be twisted. Modern manufacturing methods allow complex cross-sectional shapes to be milled.

K-file (e.g. Dentsply) instruments can be manufactured by twisting a square or triangular blank or by machining. Files with a triangular cross-section are more flexible than the equivalent-sized file with a square cross-section. Files with a triangular cross-section tend to have superior cutting characteristics and are more flexible, and hence less likely to transport the canal during preparation.

K-Flex files (Kerr, Romulus, MI, USA) are produced from a blank that is rhomboid in cross-section; this forms both cutting and non-cutting edges. The files are more flexible than an equivalent-sized K-file.

Flexofile (Maillefer: Fig. 5.28) instruments have a triangular cross-section and are manufactured from flexible stainless steel. Flexofiles are more efficient at cutting and removing dentine than an equivalent K-file, because the blade has a sharper angle and there is more room for debris. The tip of the file is non-cutting. This is an advantage when preparing curved canals, as the file is guided along the canal curvature, avoiding excessive

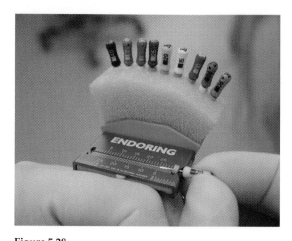

Figure 5.28

A range of Flexofile instruments. The size 20 instrument is being measured using a ruler on the Endoring.

cutting into the outer curve of the root canal or transportation. Any flexible, triangular cross-sectioned file, such as a Flexofile, can be used with the balanced force action.

Hedstroem (e.g. Dentsply: Fig. 5.29) files are machined from a tapered cylindrical block. In cross-section they have the appearance of a series of intersecting cones. Hedstroem files are highly efficient at removing dentine on the outstroke when used in a filing motion, but have poor fracture resistance in rotation.

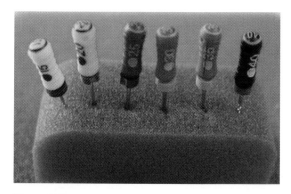

Figure 5.29

Hedstroem files.

Instruments for Coronal Flaring

The following rotary instruments are used to prepare the coronal part of the root canal before the main part is prepared by hand instruments.

Gates-Glidden Burs

These burs are used in a low-speed handpiece and are extremely efficient at removing dentine in the relatively straight parts of the root canal. They come in six sizes (Fig. 5.30) (1–6, diameters 0.5–1.5 mm) and two lengths. Penetrating too deep into curved canals can result in iatrogenic damage, e.g. a strip perforation; for this reason they must be used with care.

Nickel–Titanium Orifice Openers

These files are used to flare the coronal aspect of the root canal. Although they are manufactured from nickel–titanium the files are relatively inflexible, as the cross-sectional diameter is larger than that of a standard file. The use of these instruments is therefore best restricted to the relatively straight parts of the root canal to avoid strip perforation. It is recommended that they are used in a handpiece driven by an electric motor at 150–300 rpm (Fig. 5.31).

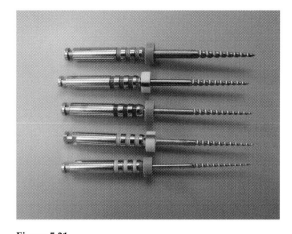

Figure 5.31

The Profile orifice openers (Dentsply).

PREPARATION TECHNIQUES

The aims of root canal preparation are:

- To remove infected debris from the root canal system
- To shape the canal allowing thorough disinfection with irrigants and intracanal medication (Fig. 5.32)
- To provide a space for the placement of a root canal filling. The filling material should ideally seal the entire root canal system from the periodontal tissues and oral cavity.

Terminology

Crown-down Preparation

The root canal system of a tooth can be prepared to give a tapered preparation in essentially two ways: apical to coronal or coronal to apical. Preparation of the coronal part of the root canal first has several significant advantages (Fig. 5.33):

1. The bulk of the infected material is found in the pulp chamber and the coronal third of the root canal system. Removal of this material early in preparation reduces the bacterial load considerably and prevents

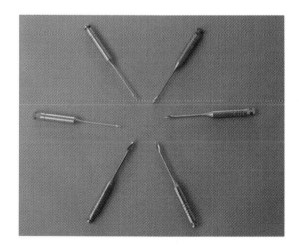

Figure 5.30

Gates-Glidden burs 1–6.

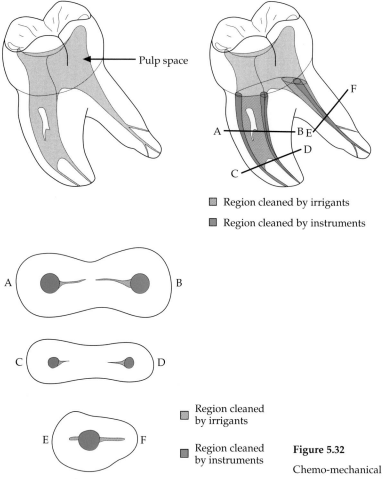

Region cleaned by irrigants

Region cleaned by instruments

Region cleaned by irrigants

Region cleaned by instruments

Figure 5.32

Chemo-mechanical preparation.

inoculation of the periapical tissues with bacteria extruded by hydraulic pressures during preparation. A file placed to the working length before coronal flaring will act like a piston in a cylinder and force material beyond the apex. Infected dentine chips and bacteria that are extruded will cause postoperative discomfort.

2. Early flaring of the coronal part of the root canal removes dentine constrictions, so that subsequent instruments do not bind short of the working length.

3. If the working length is estimated following coronal preparation then there will be little change in length during preparation. Over-preparation due to poor length control could be a cause of postoperative pain.

4. Preparing the coronal part of the root canal first enables more rapid penetration of irrigants apically. If a pool of irrigant is maintained in the access cavity then this will be guided into the root canal system during preparation. Dentine chips will be kept in suspension, thereby avoiding blockages.

Many procedural errors have been encountered when the apical portion of the root canal system has been prepared first, such as zip and elbow formation, instrument fracture, and an increased chance of postoperative

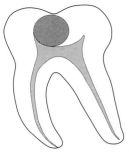

A mandibular molar with unprepared canals and carious exposure of the pulp.

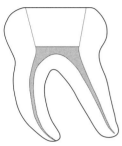

An access cavity has been prepared and the caries removed. There is straight-line vision of the canals.

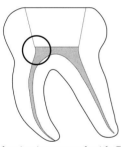

The lip of dentine is removed with Gates-Glidden burs during coronal flaring or with special ultrasonic tips, giving better straight-line access.

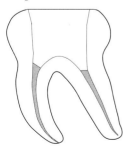

The completed access cavity.

Figure 5.33

Crown-down preparation.

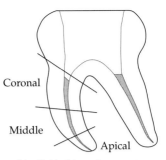

The canal is divided into three parts: coronal straight part, middle and apical.
In the distal canal in this case the coronal and apical parts converge.

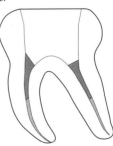

Coronal flaring is carried out using files, Gates-Glidden burs or orifice shapers.
Following coronal preparation the root length is estimated using an apex locator and a radiograph.

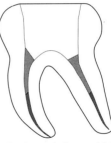

Apical preparation is carried out with hand files or rotary instruments.

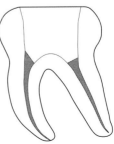

The preparation is completed, creating a gradual taper. This can be produced by stepping back with multiple instruments or by using an instrument with greater taper.

flare-up due to greater extrusion of infected debris. The outer curve of the apical part of the root canal is frequently over-prepared with filing techniques.

Procedural Errors

Transportation, Elbows and Zips

Transportation results from the selective removal of dentine from the root canal wall in a specified part. In cross-section the central point of the canal will have moved laterally. Transportation can be carried out electively (during coronal flaring to straighten the canal), or may occur as an iatrogenic error resulting from the incorrect use of hand instruments. Internal transportation is used to describe the movement of the canal system internally. External transportation occurs when the canal is over-prepared and the apical foramen is enlarged or moved; often the foramen becomes a tear-drop shape (Fig. 5.34).

Elbows and zips are caused by the file attempting to straighten in the root canal as it is worked up and down. Filing produces a canal that takes on an hourglass shape, with the narrowest cross-sectional area at the elbow and with the canal widening into the zipped region further apically. The resultant space is difficult to clean and obturate.

Strip Perforation

Strip perforation occurs in the middle part of the inner curve of a root canal if excessive dentine is removed during preparation (Fig. 5.35). This may be a result of relatively large and stiff files attempting to straighten within the root canal, or of over-use of Gates-Glidden burs or orifice shapers.

Movement of Files

Balanced Force

This is a method of preparing the root canal with hand instruments in a rotary action (see later).

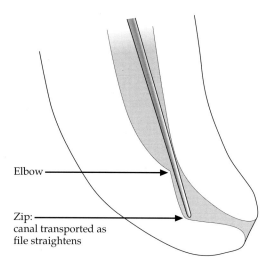

Figure 5.34

Zip and elbow.

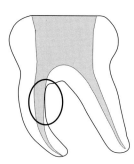

Figure 5.35

The circled area in the mesial canals is the position where a strip perforation could occur by over-preparation.

Filing

Filing consists of an apical–coronal movement of the file whilst applying lateral force against the wall of the canal. The file is moved 1–2 mm.

Hedstroem files are extremely efficient in a filing action, and cut on the outstroke.

Stainless steel files need to be precurved when filing curved canals, as the inherent restoring force in the file will attempt to straighten it within the confines of the root canal and lead to a distorted canal shape known as zipping. Nickel–titanium files should not be used in a filing motion. Even though the instruments are very flexible there will be a tendency to over-prepare the outer curve of the root canal in the apical region, as the files cannot be precurved.

Circumferential filing involves working files progressively around all the walls of the canal. It is used to ensure that the maximum area of dentine is instrumented. Over-zealous filing, however, can result in perforation. Even with overlapping file strokes it is unlikely that all the surfaces of the canal will actually be instrumented.

Anticurvature filing involves filing preferentially towards the outer curve of the root canal, away from the furcation, to avoid strip perforation. For example the buccal, mesial and lingual walls of the mesial canals of a mandibular molar would be filed more than the distal wall during coronal flaring, with more strokes on each of these walls in a ratio of 3 : 1.

Reciprocating Action

Actions such as stem-winding, watch-winding and a quarter-turn pull combine rotary and filing actions. Reciprocating actions rotate the file gently in a clockwise and counter-clockwise motion of approximately 45 degrees; the file can gradually be advanced apically. Watch-winding actions are particularly useful for exploring a tortuous canal with very fine files (ISO 06–10).

Apical Flare (or Stepping Back)

The apical part of the root canal is normally flared to facilitate filling of the canal space. Traditionally, files have been used to instrument the canal at progressively shorter lengths (0.5 to 1.0 mm) for concurrent increases in file size. This will produce an increased taper to the preparation. As stainless steel files of large diameters (>ISO size 35) become stiff, care must be used to prevent transportation in curved canals. A much more predictable method of flaring the apical preparation is by using a greater tapered instrument. These are made of nickel–titanium and need to be used with a balanced force technique. One single instrument takes the place of a series of instruments used in stepping back.

Recapitulation

Recapitulation simply means repeating again: a smaller file is passed to the working length to ensure that length has not been lost during preparation and to encourage irrigant exchange in the apical ramifications of the canal system. The use of files with greater taper makes recapitulation largely unnecessary.

Patency Maintenance

The aim of patency filing is to prevent leaving infected material in the apical 0.5–1.0 mm beyond the working length. Some endodontists advocate that small files (<ISO 10) should be passed beyond the working length and therefore potentially through the apex during preparation, to ensure that the canal is completely patent. This procedure could result in extrusion of bacteria and infected dentine chips beyond the apex, and should therefore be carried out with extreme care. Small instruments are used to displace the infected debris into the irrigant-filled canal; large sizes and vigorous filing should be avoided, as they could result in postoperative pain. If the canal is prepared to the zero reading on an apex locator then patency will normally be maintained; there is therefore no need to instrument beyond this.

Length Estimation

The length of the root canal can be estimated by using an apex locator and a confirmatory working length radiograph. It is not appropriate to try to estimate the location of the constriction in a root canal by tactile sense alone, as this too often leads to inaccurate measurements.

The Apex Locator

The apex locator (Fig. 5.36) is an electrical device that allows the operator to estimate the canal length, and with practice can be

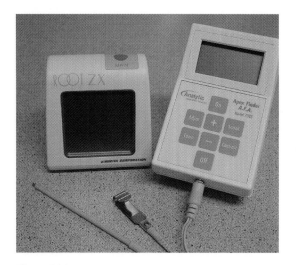

Figure 5.36

Two popular apex locators; both work using multiple frequencies and are extremely accurate.

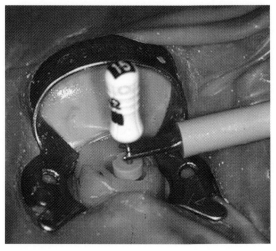

Figure 5.37

The tip of the apex locator is kept in contact with the file as it is advanced apically.

extremely accurate. Apex locators work by applying an alternating current between two electrodes; one makes contact with the lip or cheek (the ground electrode), the other is attached to a file in the root canal (Fig. 5.37). The impedance at the apical foramen is approximately equal to that between the periodontal ligament and the oral mucosa; this value is used to calibrate the instrument. The apex locator has a display showing the zero reading that indicates when the file tip is at the apical foramen. Some modern apex locators measure the impedance at two or more frequencies to improve the accuracy of the instrument. Some can be used effectively even in the presence of electrolytes such as sodium hypochlorite and blood, although these are best avoided; the pulp floor should always be dry to prevent short-circuiting.

Troubleshooting with an Apex Locator

No reading

- Is the unit switched on?
- Are the leads all connected and is the lip hook in place?
- Are the batteries fully charged?

Short reading

- Is the file short-circuiting through a metallic restoration?
- Make sure the canals and pulp chamber are relatively dry.
- Is it likely that there may be a perforation in the root?
- Is there the likelihood of a large lateral canal?
- Is there a communication between canals?—for instance, between mesiobuccal canals of maxillary first molars, or mesial canals of mandibular molars.

Long reading

- Is it possible that the apical region has been destroyed by chronic inflammatory resorption? (For instance, in cases with chronic apical periodontitis and large lesions; in these cases try a larger file.)
- Check the battery power.

Radiographic Techniques for Length Estimation

Apex locators should not take the place of working length estimation radiographs, but make an excellent adjunct for accurate identification of the root canal terminus. In this situation, when used regularly an apex locator will help reduce the number of radiographs required for endodontic treatment. The apex of the tooth is more likely to be located accurately first time by these means than with tactile methods.

Taking a good radiograph with the rubber dam and clamp in situ can be difficult; with practice, however, it becomes predictable. The Endoray (Dentsply) is particularly useful for ensuring that the X-ray beam is correctly aligned and not coned off (Fig. 5.38). The film must never be bent. Cutting down on repeat exposures reduces the radiation dose to the patient. If coronal flaring is carried out at the start of root canal preparation it should be possible to use at least a size 15 file to estimate working length. The tip of such a file can easily be viewed on radiographs.

Estimating the Working Length

If the length radiograph shows that the file tip is more than 3 mm from the apical foramen then the radiograph should be repeated (Fig. 5.39). On some occasions it may also be necessary to take more than one working length radiograph at varying angles. There is no significant difference in the ability to assess root length using digital radiography or conventional film; however, there is a significant reduction in radiation dose and time with digital radiography.

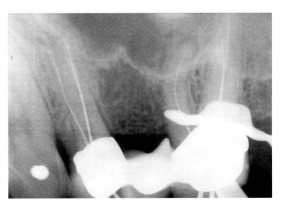

Figure 5.39

A length-estimation radiograph. The three files in the premolar were not clearly visible and a separate radiograph was taken.

Separating Root Canals in Length Estimation Radiographs

Mandibular incisors (Fig. 5.40)

Separating the buccal and lingual canals of mandibular incisors can be difficult, unless the X-ray cone is rotated by a few degrees, either left or right, to separate the canals; but care must be taken to ensure that the treated tooth is centred on the film.

Mandibular premolars

The lingual canal of a mandibular premolar can often be separated from the main (buccal) canal by aiming the beam from an anterior (and inferior) direction.

Mandibular molars (Fig. 5.41)

Separating the buccal and lingual canals of the mesial or distal roots of mandibular molars can be achieved by rotating the beam to a more anterior projection.

Maxillary premolars

Separating buccal and lingual canals can be achieved by aiming the beam from an anterior direction. If Spencer Wells forceps are used to hold the film behind the rubber dam, then it is not necessary to remove the rubber dam frame.

Maxillary molars

To separate the first and second mesiobuccal canals the cone should be aimed from the distal aspect.

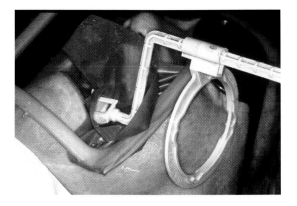

Figure 5.38

The Endoray.

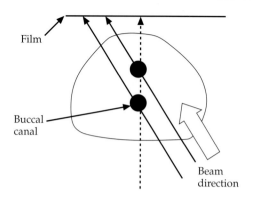

Mandibular incisor:
moving cone left or right
separates canals.

Figure 5.40

Mandibular incisors.

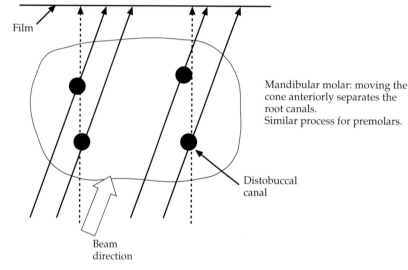

Mandibular molar: moving the
cone anteriorly separates the
root canals.
Similar process for premolars.

Figure 5.41

Mandibular molars.

HAND PREPARATION

It is exacting and time-consuming to learn a new technique and become conversant with it. Practice on extracted teeth is invaluable before embarking on the treatment of a patient.

Crown-down Preparation

The principles of crown-down preparation will be described. This allows the practitioner to develop a personalized technique that follows the ideals of modern crown-down preparation without unnecessary detail.

Rationale

The root canal is divided into three parts: the coronal 'straight' part of the root canal, the apical part, and a middle part termed the 'merging' part.

Coronal Preparation

The coronal part of the root canal is prepared first. As it is relatively straight the instruments used to prepare it do not have to be very flexible. A combination of files, Gates-Glidden burs and nickel–titanium orifice openers can be used. The depth to which initial preparation is carried out should be estimated from the preoperative radiograph.

The canal must be irrigated throughout preparation to remove debris, kill microbes and prevent blocking. The use of files before Gates-Glidden burs can be used to transport the orifice of a canal deliberately. This decreases the initial curvature of the canal and improves straight-line access. The burs should be used in a planing action, cutting against the thickest wall of the root canal as the drill is withdrawn from the canal. Applying apical pressure and drilling into the root canal should be avoided, as this can lead to over-enlargement and ledging.

Apical Preparation

This will involve preparation around a curve in the vast majority of canals, and is the region in which most iatrogenic errors have occurred in the past. Once the coronal part of the root canal has been prepared, access to the apical part is made easier. Instruments used to prepare the apical part of the root canal system need to be thin and flexible, and are made of materials such as flexible stainless steel or nickel–titanium.

Before apical preparation is started an estimate of the root canal length must be made, ideally using an apex locator and confirmed with a radiograph.

If coronal preparation has been carried out, then there will be less change in the length of the preparation during instrumentation. The lengths are marked on the file with a rubber stop to a clearly definable and easily remembered reference point, which is best recorded in the patient's notes.

The size of the apical preparation and master apical file will depend on:

1. The size of the natural canal.
2. The obturation technique that is to be used (with vertically compacted warm techniques the apical termination of the preparation should be kept as small as practicable).
3. The overall taper of the root canal.

The apex is prepared to the working length with a file of not less than ISO size 25, as this allows delivery of irrigant to the most apical part of the root canal system. Irrigant can be carried apically and replenished by recapitulation with files.

Using the Balanced Force Action for Apical Preparation

The balanced force action when used with flexible files results in a more centred preparation and less transportation than with a filing technique.

The technique (Roane et al 1985)
This instrumentation technique uses clockwise/anticlockwise rotational motion to remove dentine with flexible stainless steel files or nickel–titanium files (Fig. 5.42). It is useful for rapidly removing dentine in curved canals whilst maintaining curvature (files are not precurved).

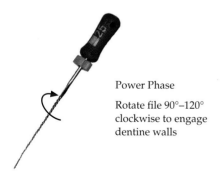

Power Phase

Rotate file 90°–120° clockwise to engage dentine walls

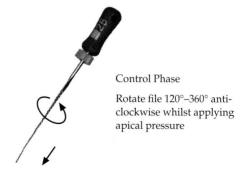

Control Phase

Rotate file 120°–360° anti-clockwise whilst applying apical pressure

Figure 5.42

The Balanced Force action.

- Place the file into the canal until light resistance is met and turn it up to 90°–120° clockwise to engage the dentine walls (the power phase).
- Whilst applying light apical pressure (to prevent the file backing out of the canal) turn 120°–360° anticlockwise. Listen for a 'click' as a bite of dentine is removed (the control phase).
- Repeat the clockwise/anticlockwise motion until the file reaches the desired length. If the file does not appear to be cutting, then it should be rotated clockwise to load the flutes with debris and removed for cleaning. Check the instrument for damage; discard if evident.

Some instruments (e.g. Greater Taper files: Dentsply) are ground in the reverse direction and will therefore need to be used in the opposite manner.

Using Greater Taper Files for Apical Preparation

Greater Taper files are manufactured from nickel–titanium and have to be used with a reverse balanced force action (Fig. 5.43). To prevent the tip binding and possibly fracturing it is important to prepare a pilot channel (glide path) for the instruments to follow. The canal is instrumented to the working length using a balanced force action with Flexofiles to at least a size 25. Greater Taper files can then be worked to the same length instead of stepping back with multiple instruments.

The different tapers may be appropriate for different situations (Table 5.3).

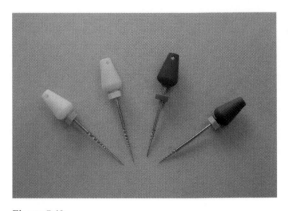

Figure 5.43

Greater Taper hand files: white 0.06, yellow 0.08, red 0.10, blue 0.12.

Merging

The apical and coronal preparation should merge into one another in a gradual smooth taper. This can often be achieved with a single Greater Taper instrument, as opposed to stepping back with multiple instruments.

Crown-down Preparation Techniques

The following crown-down hand preparation techniques are described:

- Stepdown
- Modified Double Flare

Table 5.3 *Tapers appropriate for various root canal situations*

Colour	Taper	Use
White	0.06	All thin or narrow canals.
Yellow	0.08	Multicanal premolars, mesial roots of mandibular molars, buccal roots of maxillary molars.
Red	0.10	Palatal canal of maxillary molars, distal roots of mandibular molars, single-rooted premolars, mandibular canines and maxillary anteriors.
Blue	0.12	Large straight canals and canals with large terminal diameter.

Stepdown Technique of Canal Preparation

(A hand-filing technique with precurved files: Goerig et al (1982).)

Precurving Files

Files can be easily and accurately precurved in a file-bending device (Fig. 5.44). The curve is estimated from the radiograph, and by feedback from small files that are placed in the canal at the start of treatment.

Initial Coronal Flare

Insert a size 15 Hedstroem file into the straight part of the root canal (16 mm from cusp tips in a typical molar). Pull back in a filing motion and repeat, with more strokes on the outer curved wall than the inner wall, until the file is loose. Irrigate with hypochlorite. Repeat with sizes 20 and 25.

Insert a Gates-Glidden bur size 1 into the straight part of the canal; plane the outer wall gently in an apical–coronal direction. Repeat with sizes 2 and 3 to shorter distances. Use copious irrigation or waterspray to prevent clogging the canals with dentine chips.

Apical Preparation

Insert a fine Flexofile, such as size 10 or 15, 0.5–1.0 mm short of the apical constriction. This is verified with an apex locator and radiograph. *Files are precurved* to conform to the

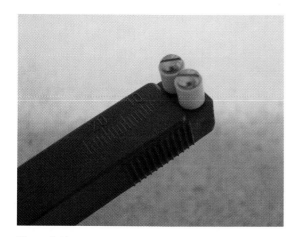

Figure 5.44

A Flexobend for precurving files.

canal shape. Pull the file back in a filing motion. Reinsert and repeat, working around the canal walls until the file is loose. Irrigate. Repeat with the next largest file up to size 25.

Apical Flare (Stepback)

A Greater Taper instrument is selected and used with a reverse balanced force action to flare the apical preparation. It is no longer necessary to use a sequence of instruments to step back.

The Modified Double-Flare Technique

(A technique that uses the balanced force instrumentation action: Saunders and Saunders (1992).)

Coronal Preparation

Check the length of the straight section of the coronal part of the root canal from a preoperative radiograph. Take a size 35 or 40 file with the stop set at this length, coat with lubricant and instrument with balanced force action to the full length of the straight part of the canal. If a size 35 is too tight then a smaller instrument will need to be used.

Continue to prepare the straight part of the canal with hand files until a size 1 Gates-Glidden bur will fit in the canal. A size 40 instrument will create a canal with an orifice diameter of at least 0.5 mm and should provide sufficient space. Irrigate between files.

Use Gates-Glidden burs 1, 2 and 3 cutting on outward stroke to flare the canal, being careful not to over-prepare. Use copious irrigation with Gates-Glidden burs.

Preparation of the Apical Section

A size 10 file should now pass just short of the full working length. Use a size 15 file to instrument to the estimated working length using balanced force action. Length is verified with an apex locator and confirmed with a radiograph.

The canal is then prepared to the working length with increasing file sizes to a master apical file (MAF) of 35–40 using balanced force. The size of the MAF will depend on the size of the original canal and the degree of curvature. Fine, severely curved canals may only be prepared to the minimum size (ISO 25). Irrigate between each file.

Apical Flaring (Stepping Back)

This can be achieved with a Greater Taper file, as already described.

Troubleshooting Preparation of Root Canals

Transportation

Precurving files reduces the restoring force that is applied to the root canal wall, and consequently reduces the chance of transportation. Using the balanced force instrumentation technique with non-end cutting, flexible files will produce less transportation of the canal.

Ledges can also be created with Gates-Glidden burs during coronal flaring; this can be avoided if the bur is used to plane the wall of the root canal as it is withdrawn, rather than being forced apically as if drilling down the root canal.

Perforation

Perforation is the iatrogenic damage to the tooth or root canal wall that results in a connection being made with the periodontal ligament or oral cavity.

Perforation can be avoided by:

1. Using the pulp floor map to locate root canal orifices
2. Gradually working up the series from small files to larger sizes, always recapitulating with a smaller file between sizes
3. Using an apex locator and radiograph to confirm root canal length
4. Minimizing overuse of Gates-Glidden burs, either too deep or too large, in curved canals where a strip perforation may occur. Try and direct the cutting action into the bulkiest wall of dentine; this also helps straighten the first curvature of the root canal and improves straight-line access.
5. Restricting the use of 'orifice openers' to small sizes in narrow canals
6. Using an anticurvature filing technique to remove dentine selectively from the bulkiest wall
7. Never forcing instruments or jumping sizes
8. Irrigating copiously; not only will this disinfect the root canal and dissolve organic material, but it will also keep dentine chips in suspension and prevent blocking. If dentine chips are packed into the apical region of the root canal then the preparation can become transported internally. This could eventually lead to perforation.

Blockage

Blockage can be avoided by:

1. Using copious amounts of irrigant. This will keep dentine chips suspended in the irrigant so that they can be flushed from the root canal system during preparation. Solutions such as EDTA are particularly useful, as they act as chelating agents, causing clumping together of particles.
2. Keeping the pulp chamber flooded with irrigant during preparation; this allows the continuous transfer and replenishment of irrigant within the root canal system as each new file is introduced. Dentine chips are carried out into the access cavity in suspension for aspiration.

What To Do If Blockage Occurs

If a blockage occurs suddenly during root canal preparation, place a small amount of EDTA lubricant (Fig. 5.45) on a fine precurved file (ISO 10) (Fig. 5.46) and introduce it into the root canal. Use a gentle watch-winding action to work loose the dentine chips of the blockage. When patency is regained, irrigate the canal with sodium hypochlorite. This will flush out the dentine chips (effervescence may possibly help in the process). Whatever happens do not try to force instruments through a blockage; this will simply compact the dentine chips further and make the situation worse. If the blockage is persistent, endosonics may help to dislodge the dentine chips. Ultrasonic irrigation systems used at low power with full irrigant flow can sometimes dislodge blockages by the

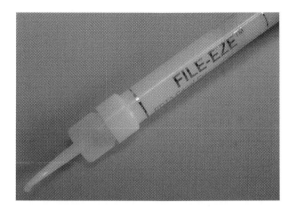

Figure 5.45

File-eze is an EDTA-based lubricant.

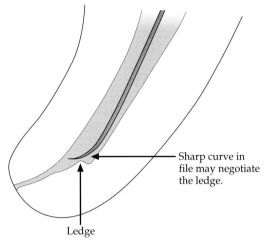

Sharp curve in file may negotiate the ledge.

Ledge

Figure 5.47

Passing ledges and blockages.

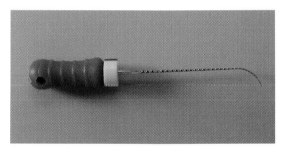

Figure 5.46

A sharp curve in a small file can be used to negotiate past blockages.

action of acoustic microstreaming around a vibrating file. Another method to bypass a ledge is to put a sharp curve at the tip of the file so that it overcomes the defect (Fig. 5.47).

Fractured Instrument

Unfortunately the occasional instrument may fracture unexpectedly; but this should be a rare occurrence. Fracture (or separation, as it is sometimes euphemistically called) is perhaps more frequent with nickel–titanium instruments. The risk of instrument fracture can be reduced by:

1. Always progressing through the sizes of files in sequence, and not jumping sizes. Forcing an instrument will inevitably lead to fracture.

2. Discarding all damaged files. Any that are overwound or unwound should be discarded, as should those that have been used in very tightly curved canals.
3. Taking particular care with nickel–titanium files. The files should be used for only a limited number of times and then discarded.
4. Not rotating Hedstroem files.

Loss of Length

Length of preparation can be lost if dentine chips are compacted into the apical part of the root canal system during preparation. This occurs if the root canal is devoid of irrigant. When patency is lost the canal may be transported. A crown-down technique will help to reduce the chances of this happening by allowing more irrigant into the canal during preparation; the use of lubricant may also prevent packing of dentine chips.

Over-preparation

Over-preparation can be avoided by restricting use to smaller instruments. Over-flaring coronally should be avoided, as strip perforation can occur in the danger areas of a root canal system and the tooth is unnecessarily weakened, compromising subsequent restoration.

Wine-bottle Effect (Fig. 5.48)

Not the consequence of drinking too much, but the shape that is created from overuse of Gates-Glidden burs to flare coronally! The wine-bottle effect can make obturation difficult, will increase the risk of strip perforation and weakens the tooth.

These problems will be avoided if Gates-Glidden burs are used sequentially to plane the walls of the root canal, and larger sizes are used to progressively shorter distances, or they are sustituted by orifice openers.

MECHANICAL PREPARATION TECHNIQUES

Introduction

Rotary endodontic instruments manufactured from nickel–titanium are 3–4 times more flexible than equivalent flexible stainless steel instruments. The instruments have a greater taper than standard instruments (0.02 mm per mm),

while retaining flexibility. Modern mechanically driven instruments are designed for use in a continuous rotary action at a slow speed (150–350 rpm). They have been shown to produce little transportation of the root canal. There are now many different systems available, but the basic principles for their use are similar.

Basic Principles of Use

Rotation

The use of a torque-controlled electric motor and a speed-reducing handpiece (Fig. 5.49) is more reliable than a handpiece fitted to an airmotor. It is much more difficult to control the speed of air-driven handpieces predictably, and therefore their use can lead to instrument fracture.

Speed

It is important that the instruments are used at the manufacturer's recommended speed. Most rotary files should be rotated at speeds

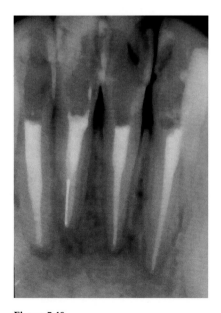

Figure 5.48

Over-use of Gates-Glidden burs in these mandibular incisors has resulted in a wine-bottle effect.

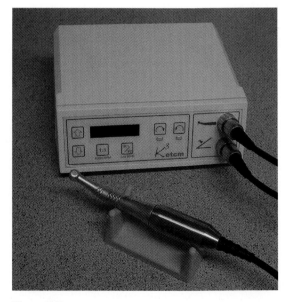

Figure 5.49

An electric motor and speed-reducing handpiece is essential for rotary preparation techniques.

between 150 and 350 rpm for routine root canal preparation.

Cutting Action

The instruments should be advanced into the canal with a light apical–coronal action (pecking/pumping) in waves of 8–10 seconds. They are then withdrawn, assessed for damage, cleaned of debris and reinserted. Files must be kept moving coronally–apically within the canal; rotating an instrument at a stationary position close to or at full working length results in alternating compression and strain in the file at the greatest point of its curvature, and could eventually lead to instrument failure. The root canals are flooded with irrigant or lubricant during instrumentation to prevent dentine chips compacting. Packing of dentine chips around the file can lead to binding and instrument fracture.

Canal Curvature

Nickel–titanium, because of its superelasticity, can be rotated in canals of sharp curvature; but care must be taken in severely curved canals. In very curved canals or canals with sudden abrupt apical curvatures hand instrumentation is preferred for completion of preparation.

Avoidance of Instrument Fracture

To avoid fracture it is important to create a pilot channel that the non-cutting tip of a rotary instrument can follow. If such a channel is not created the tip may bind and fracture.

Preparation should be carried out in a crown-down manner, as this ensures that successive instruments are not overworked.

Nickel–titanium instruments can fracture unpredictably, and may not show signs of permanent deformation before failing. Instruments should therefore be changed regularly and should never be forced during preparation. It is often recommended that nickel–titanium instruments should not be used in more than 5–10 canals.

The Instruments

There are two basic types:

For Coronal Preparation

Orifice openers are usually relatively thick in diameter and are consequently not very flexible. They are designed for coronal flaring, and should only be used in the 'straight' part of a root canal.

For Apical Preparation

Tapered rotary files are available in tapers of 0.04, 0.06, 0.08, 0.10 and 0.12. Profiles (Dentsply), Quantec (Analytic Endodontics, Glendora, CA, USA), Hero (Micro-mega, Geneva, Switzerland), K3 (Kerr, Bretton, Peterborough, UK) and Greater Taper files are essentially used to flare rapidly a preprepared pilot channel in the apical part of the root canal. Instruments are used in a crown-down manner (Figs. 5.50–5.53).

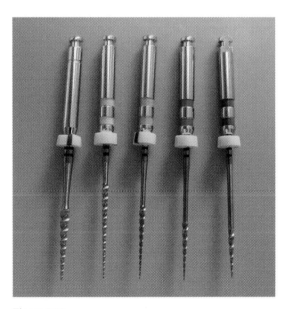

Figure 5.50

The Greater Taper rotary range of instruments: an accessory file for coronal flaring (left) and then tapers 0.06, 0.08, 0.10, 0.12.

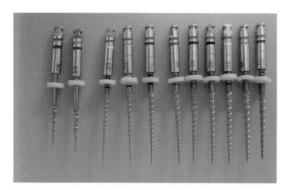

Figure 5.51

K3 rotary instruments. The first two on the left are used for coronal flaring; the others can be used apically.

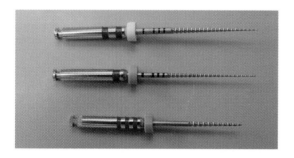

Figure 5.52

Profiles: orifice openers have three bands, 0.06 tapers two bands and 0.04 tapers a single band.

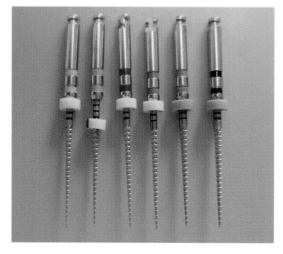

Figure 5.53

A range of Profile 0.06 taper instruments.

Root Canal Preparation with Rotary Instruments

The aim of preparation is to produce a gradually tapering shape in the bulk of the root canal system, with the narrowest diameter apically, the greatest diameter coronally and a smooth flow between the two. The apical preparation must be at least an ISO size 25 to allow good irrigant penetration.

Divide the canal mentally into three parts:
Coronal ('Straight part of canal')
Middle ('Merging')
Apical ('Apical preparation')

Coronal Preparation

Nickel–titanium orifice openers are relatively inflexible and are therefore only suitable for use in the coronal 'straight part' part of the root canal. This distance can be estimated from the pre-treatment radiograph. The canal should be irrigated between instruments using sodium hypochlorite solution.

The canal is first instrumented using Flexofiles sizes 10–40 in a balanced force action within the coronal 'straight' part of the root canal. This can be estimated from the preoperative diagnostic radiograph. Orifice openers are then used in sequence to flare the canal rapidly to the same length. They can be used in ascending or descending order. A larger instrument will make room for a smaller instrument, allowing deeper penetration.

Where the canal is already greater than an ISO size 40, orifice openers can be used without the necessity of preparing a pilot channel.

Apical Preparation

Following coronal preparation the root canal length is measured using an apex locator (zero reading) and confirmed with a radiograph. The working length should be 0–1 mm from the root canal terminus. A pilot channel is prepared using stainless steel hand instruments to the working length; this acts as a guide for the nickel–titanium instruments.

Preparation of the Pilot Channel

The pilot channel is prepared using Flexofiles sizes 15–25 with the balanced force technique (see hand instrumentation). The canal is irrigated with hypochlorite solution between instruments, and in fine canals an EDTA-based lubricant may also be used to prevent binding of instruments and compaction of any dentine chips that may have been created.

The canal can now be flared to the desired taper. Nickel–titanium instruments are rotated at 150–350 rpm in a speed-reducing handpiece using an electric torque-controlled motor. Instruments should be used sequentially. The master apical size must be at least size 25 for good irrigant penetration.

Middle Section of the Canal: 'Merging'

If apical instrumentation has been completed with a smaller-taper instrument (0.02, 0.04), the coronal and apical preparation may need to be merged by using an instrument with a larger taper. This will create a smooth flow to the preparation.

During mechanical preparation the canal is thoroughly irrigated with sodium hypochlorite solution. This can be carried out with hand syringes or endosonic handpieces.

FURTHER READING

Buchanan LS (2000). The standardized-taper root canal preparation—Part 1. Concepts for variably tapered shaping instruments. *International Endodontic Journal* **33:** 516–529.

Goerig AC, Michelich RJ, Schultz HH (1982). Instrumentation of root canals in molar using the step-down technique. *Journal of Endodontics* **8:** 550–554.

Roane JB, Sabala CL, Duncanson MG (1985). The 'balanced force' concept for instrumentation of curved canals. *Journal of Endodontics* **11:** 203–211.

Saunders WP, Saunders EM (1992). Effect of non-cutting tipped instruments on the quality of root canal preparation using a modified double-flared technique. *Journal of Endodontics* **18:** 32–36.

Schilder H (1974). Cleaning and shaping the root canal. *Dental Clinics of North America* **18:** 269–296.

European Society of Endodontology (1994). Consensus report of the European Society of Endodontology on quality guidelines for endodontic treatment. *International Endodontic Journal* **27:** 115–124.

6 IRRIGATION AND MEDICATION

CONTENTS • Why? • Irrigants • How? • Medicaments • Further Reading

WHY?

Following thorough instrumentation of an infected root canal there will be a significantly reduced number of bacteria present; but it is well documented that instrumentation alone cannot clean all the internal surfaces of the root canal. Bacteria can be found on the root canal walls, within dentine tubules and in lateral canals. Antibacterial irrigants and inter-appointment medicaments are needed to kill the remaining micro-organisms.

A large series of follow up studies have shown that, by using thorough mechanical preparation, irrigation with sodium hypochlorite and dressing with calcium hydroxide, predictable disinfection can be achieved in almost 100% of root canals. This in turn has produced clinical and radiographic evidence of healing apical periodontitis in over 90% of cases.

Medicaments are also invaluable in preventing the recolonization of the root canal between appointments. If the canal space is left empty then the small number of bacteria remaining can multiply to levels equivalent to those that were initially present.

IRRIGANTS

Irrigants should:

- Be antimicrobial
- Have a low surface tension
- Not be mutagenic, carcinogenic or overtly cytotoxic
- Possess tissue-dissolving properties
- Aid the removal of smear layer
- Remain active following storage
- Be inexpensive.

Preparations Used as Irrigants

Sodium Hypochlorite

Sodium hypochlorite solution has been used as an irrigant in endodontics for many years. It is inexpensive, readily available, and highly antimicrobial, and has valuable tissue-dissolving properties. A 0.5% solution kills bacteria. Sodium hypochlorite solutions greater than 1% will effectively dissolve organic tissue. Solutions ranging in strength from 0.5% to 5.25% have been recommended for use in endodontics (Fig. 6.1). Increasing the concentration will increase the rate at which organic material is dissolved, and may improve its effectiveness as an antibacterial agent. Heating the solution will have a similar effect (Fig. 6.2). The tissue-dissolving ability of sodium hypochlorite is affected by the amount of organic material present in the canal, the fluid flow and the surface area available.

The volume of solution used is probably more important than the concentration. Several millilitres should be exchanged frequently throughout the root canal system during instrumentation. Frequent replenishment will improve the flushing action of the irrigant, which removes debris. Keeping the canal system flooded with fresh solution at all times during preparation will improve dissolution of organic material and killing of

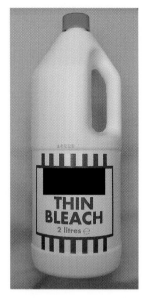

Figure 6.1

Household thin bleach is a readily available sodium hypochlorite solution. It is important to check that there are no additives such as perfumes or sodium hydroxide.

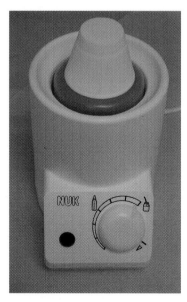

Figure 6.2

A baby-bottle warmer is probably the easiest means of heating hypochlorite solution. Prolonged heating will inactivate the solution.

bacteria. Rubber dam is essential for endodontic treatment, and will prevent the leaking of sodium hypochlorite solution into the patient's mouth; the patient's clothes should be protected with a bib. Using a safe-ended needle can prevent extrusion of sodium hypochlorite into the periapical tissues.

Saline

The use of saline as the sole irrigant is not considered appropriate, as normal solutions are ineffective as antimicrobial agents and will not dissolve organic material.

Local Anaesthetic

Local anaesthetic should not be used as the sole irrigant, as it has no advantages over normal saline, which is not considered effective.

Chlorhexidine Gluconate

Chlorhexidine gluconate can be purchased as a mouthwash in a 0.2% solution. Chlorhexidine, while antibacterial, will not dissolve organic material, and is also relatively expensive. It may be effective in concentrations from 0.2–2.0%, but there is little published clinical evidence.

Iodine in Potassium Iodide

There have been reports that some strains of bacteria that are associated with failed root canal treatment have survived in the presence of calcium hydroxide – for example, *Enterococcus faecalis*. This bacterium is susceptible to iodine in potassium iodide, and therefore this solution may be useful as an irrigant in retreatment cases. It is used as a 2% solution of iodine in 4% aqueous potassium iodide (Fig. 6.3).

EDTA (Ethylene diaminetetraacetate) (Fig. 6.4)

This is a chelating agent, and will dissolve dentine chips within the root canal system. It is not antibacterial, and will not dissolve

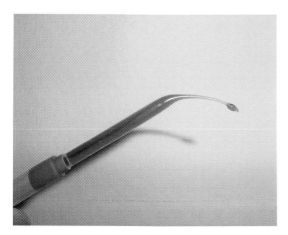

Figure 6.3

Iodine in potassium iodide solution can be used as an irrigant. Here it is applied using a dropper.

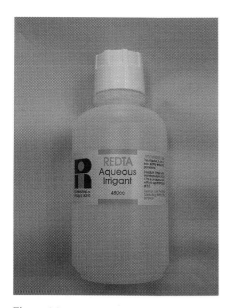

Figure 6.4

EDTA solution.

necrotic tissue or remove superficial debris; but it is very effective for removing the smear layer. It is usually purchased as a 17% solution with a pH of 8.0. When used in series with sodium hypochlorite the smear layer can be removed, allowing penetration of the

antibacterial irrigant deeper into infected dentine tubules. A final flush of the prepared root canal system with 5–10 ml of EDTA over five minutes followed by sodium hypochlorite is an effective way of removing the organic and inorganic matter from the root canal system.

Citric Acid

Citric acid has been used in periodontal treatment for conditioning root surfaces. This acid is an alternative to EDTA for removing smear layer from within the root canal system; but it probably has little advantage.

HOW?

Delivery of Irrigants

Syringe

Commercial endodontic syringes have a fine bore to allow delivery of irrigant into the apical part of the root canal system. Gauge 27 needles are manufactured with a cut away tip to allow irrigant to pass out sideways and reduce the risk of apical extrusion (Figs. 6.5–6.11).

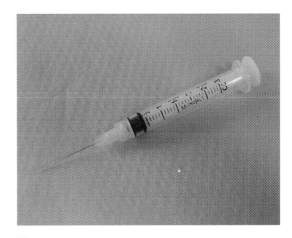

Figure 6.5

A Monoject syringe, which has a safe-ended tip.

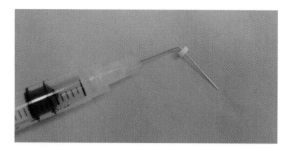

Figure 6.6

Placing a rubber stop on the needle will prevent extrusion of irrigant beyond the apex of the tooth

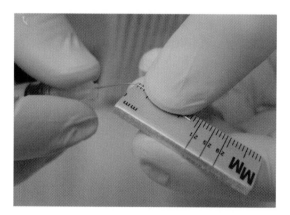

Figure 6.7

Prebending the needle against a ruler.

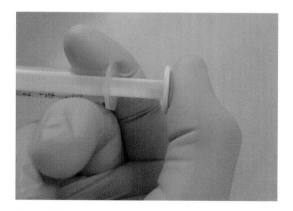

Figure 6.8

Squeezing the plunger with the thumb may result in more rapid delivery of irrigant and possible extrusion of irrigant.

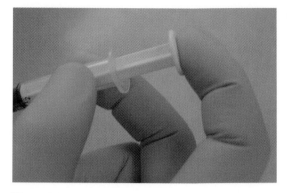

Figure 6.9

Using a forefinger to depress the plunger gives greater control of irrigant delivery.

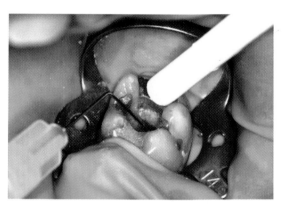

Figure 6.10

Hand irrigation in a mandibular molar.

Endosonics

Endosonics is a very useful means of delivering irrigant.

Most portable ultrasonic units can be fitted with an endosonic attachment that allows the delivery of irrigant (Fig. 6.12). During ultrasonic vibration of an endosonic file in the root canal, streaming of the irrigant is created, and this may help dislodge material from the canal system. It also ensures penetration of irrigant into lateral canals, fins and anastomoses, where files cannot penetrate. Ultrasonic streaming occurs best when a small file (size 15) is vibrated freely within the root canal (Fig. 6.13). Binding of the file

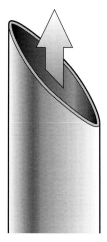
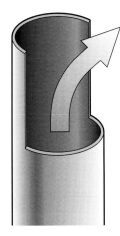
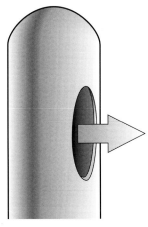

Bevelled needle: irrigant forced apically; there is a risk of extrusion if the needle becomes lodged in the canal.

Monoject tip: irrigant can pass sideways.

Safe-ended tip: irrigant passes sideways.

Figure 6.11

Endodontic needles are manufactured with a cut-away tip to allow irrigant to pass out sideways and reduce the risk of apical extrusion.

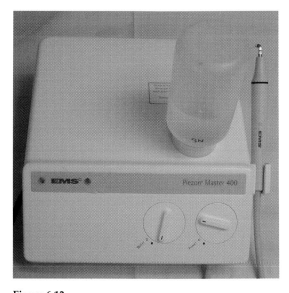

Figure 6.12

The Piezon unit (EMS, Forestgate, Dallas, TX, USA) with an endosonic insert and irrigant bottle.

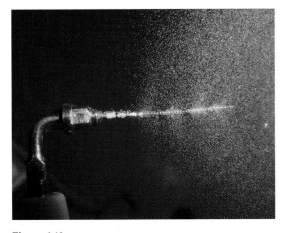

Figure 6.13

The ultrasonically energized file creates currents of streaming of irrigant within the root canal. Nodes can be seen along this file as it vibrates in air.

results in a decrease in streaming. The endosonic file should be moved up and down to facilitate irrigation and prevent possible ledging of the canal wall (Fig. 6.14). A high volume of irrigant can be exchanged with the use of endosonics (Fig. 6.15). Ultrasonic irrigation will eliminate bacteria from infected root canals more effectively than syringe irrigation alone.

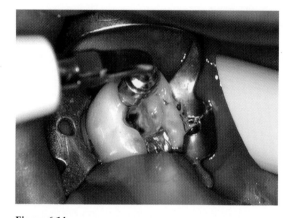

Figure 6.14

The endosonic tip in use. The aspirator tip should be kept away from the access cavity to allow irrigant to flow into the pulp canal space.

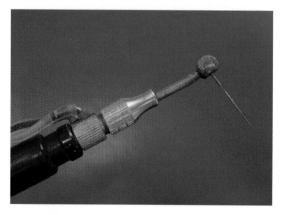

Figure 6.15

The Cavi-endo endosonic insert (Dentsply, Weybridge, Surrey, UK) . Distilled water should be run through the unit after every use to prevent corrosion damage by the sodium hypochlorite solution.

MEDICAMENTS

Why?

Intracanal medicaments are advocated to:

- Eliminate bacteria after chemomechanical instrumentation
- Reduce inflammation of the periapical tissues
- Dissolve remaining organic material
- Counteract coronal microleakage.

When?

Vital Cases

There is good evidence that in the absence of bacterial infection of the pulp space there is rarely any inflammation of the apical pulp stump or periapically. In vital cases where root canal treatment is carried out under aseptic conditions an intracanal medicament is not required. Indeed, treatment may be undertaken in a single visit.

Infected Teeth

It has been shown in clinical studies that approximately 50% of infected root canals were not disinfected using an antibacterial irrigant alone during root canal treatment. Residual bacteria remaining in the root canal following preparation are able to multiply rapidly between appointments if the canal remains empty. Antibacterial medicaments are used between appointments to kill the few remaining bacteria and prevent re-infection of the root canal. Agents such as calcium hydroxide have been shown to be highly effective. The agent used must have a wide antibacterial spectrum, and should remain active for the period between appointments. Some agents that are toxic to bacteria may damage the periapical tissues if extruded from the root canal system.

How?

The properties of an intracanal medicament:

- The antibacterial activity should be greater than the cytotoxic effect.
- The agent should be in contact with the residual bacteria.
- The agent must be present in sufficient concentration.
- Antibacterial intracanal medicaments must have a wide spectrum of activity.
- The agent must have a sufficient duration of action.

Intracanal Medicaments

Calcium Hydroxide

Calcium hydroxide is antibacterial owing to its high pH. It can be easily inserted into the prepared root canal as a thick paste, and physically restricts bacterial recolonization (Fig. 6.16). Calcium hydroxide, when placed in the root canal for at least 7 days, has been shown effectively to kill most of the pathogens found within the confines of the root canal system, and can be recommended as an antibacterial medicament. Calcium hydroxide will aid the dissolution of organic material remaining in the root canal after preparation. Calcium hydroxide has been shown experimentally to be superior to camphorated paramonochlorophenol, camphor-

ated phenol, 2% idodine–potasssium iodide, polyantimicrobials and antibiotic/steroid pastes. The medicament is easily removed from the root canal system prior to obturation using EDTA and sodium hypochlorite irrigants.

Iodine in Potassium Iodide

Iodine is a potent antibacterial agent, but has low toxicity. Iodoform pastes can be used as a medicament in refractory cases. There is a paucity of evidence for their effectiveness as a root canal medicament, and they may have a short duration of action. There are commercially available preparations such as Vitapex (Fig. 6.17). Some patients are allergic to iodine compounds, which can act as haptens.

Corticosteroid/Antibiotic Paste

These are basically antibiotic-containing pastes (Fig. 6.18). Scientifically they have been shown to be no better than calcium hydroxide as a medicament, and commercially available

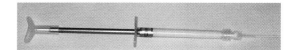

Figure 6.17

An iodoform-based medicament. This may be particularly useful in difficult retreatment cases.

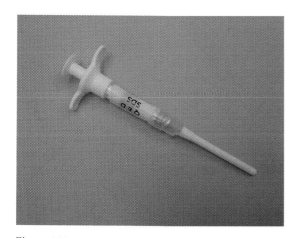

Figure 6.16

Calcium hydroxide paste in a syringe.

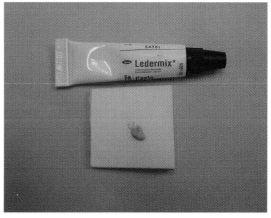

Figure 6.18

A corticosteroid/antibiotic paste.

preparations tend to be more expensive. Mixing the paste with calcium hydroxide has been advocated, but this gives little advantage and may decrease the effectiveness of the individual components, as there is no synergism between the separate materials.

Formaldehydes, Paraformaldehydes, Phenols, Camphorated Phenol, Camphorated Paramonochlorophenol

These materials have potential mutagenic and carcinogenic properties, and can become widely distributed in the body. The effectiveness of vapour-forming solutions decreases too rapidly after insertion, and contact with tissue fluids renders them inactive. The use of any of these materials can no longer be justified.

Placement of Medicaments

Syringe Delivery

Probably the easiest way of applying a medicament. Calcium hydroxide preparations come in different concentrations and in different formats. Disposable plastic tips are excellent, as there is no risk of cross-infection (Fig. 6.19). Metal syringe tips must be autoclaved between patients. It is important to place a fine file along the bore of the needle to ensure that the tip does not become blocked.

The syringe tips on most commercial systems can be pre-measured to prevent extrusion (Fig. 6.20).

Hand File

A file can be used to place the medicament in the canal. The agent should be smeared on the walls of the root canals, and can be carried to the working length by gently rotating the file in an anti-clockwise direction (Fig. 6.21). If it is mixed to a thick paste consistency a plug-

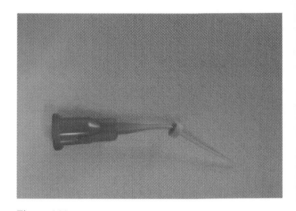

Figure 6.20

Bending the needle tip or placing a rubber stop will prevent extrusion of the medicament.

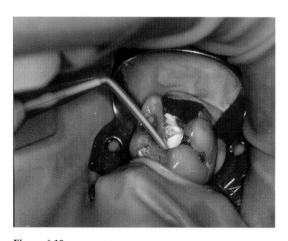

Figure 6.19

Using a needle to deliver calcium hydroxide paste into the root canals.

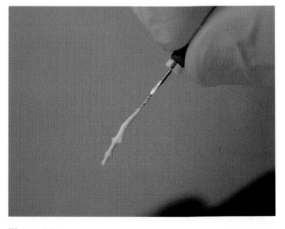

Figure 6.21

Calcium hydroxide can be placed using a file. The stop indicates the working length; medicament should coat the entire canal.

ger can be used to ensure that the material is carried completely to all parts of the prepared root canal system.

Spiral Fillers

Great care must be exercised when using spiral fillers, as the instrument can bind in the canal and fracture (Fig. 6.22); the direction of rotation must be verified before use. It is perhaps easiest to use spiral fillers by hand; but they do not really offer any great benefit over applying medicament with a hand instrument.

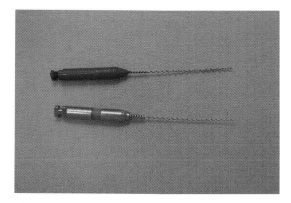

Figure 6.22

Spiral fillers.

Calcium Hydroxide Points

Calcium hydroxide-containing points are available. They are not considered to be very effective, as little calcium hydroxide is released into the root canal (Fig. 6.23).

FURTHER READING

Byström A, Sundqvist G (1981). Bacteriologic evaluation of the efficacy of mechanical root canal instrumentation in endodontic therapy. *Scandinavian Journal of Dental Research* **89:** 321–328.

Byström A, Sundqvist G (1983). Bacteriologic evaluation of the effect of 0.5 per cent sodium hypochlorite in endodontic therapy. *Oral Surgery, Oral Medicine, Oral Pathology* **55:** 307–312.

Byström A, Claesson R, Sundqvist G (1985). The antibacterial effect of camphorated paramonochlorophenol, camphorated phenol and calcium hydroxide in the treatment of infected root canals. *Endodontics and Dental Traumatology* **1:** 170–175.

Chong BS, Pitt Ford TR (1992). The role of intracanal medication in root canal treatment. *International Endodontic Journal* **25:** 97–106.

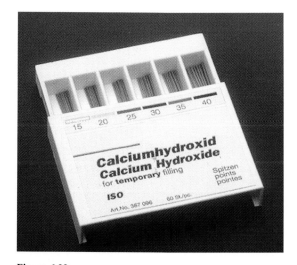

Figure 6.23

Calcium hydroxide points.

7 OBTURATION TECHNIQUES

CONTENTS • **Introduction** • **Criteria for Obturation** • **Sealers** • **Root Filling Materials** • **Obturation Techniques** • **Troubleshooting Obturation Techniques** • **Further Reading**

INTRODUCTION

Following through cleaning and shaping, the root canal system is obturated to:

- Prevent the ingress of micro-organisms into the root canal system by coronal leakage.
- Prevent the multiplication of micro-organisms remaining in the root canal system.
- Prevent percolation of tissue fluid into pulp space via apical foramina/lateral canals or furcal canals. This fluid could act as a substrate for any viable bacteria remaining following root canal treatment.
- Prevent bacterial percolation into the pulp canal space via interconnections with the gingival sulcus or periodontal pockets.

Many materials have been suggested as suitable root canal fillings; however the current material of choice is gutta percha used with a sealer.

CRITERIA FOR OBTURATION

Historically, obturation of the root canal space was often delayed until there were signs of periapical healing, and a reduction in the patient's symptoms. Delaying obturation, however, can lead to problems: if a temporary restoration fails to seal the coronal aspect of the root canal system then bacteria will enter the canal by coronal microleakage and the patient's symptoms may persist or become worse. Endodontically treated teeth can be vulnerable to fracture, and when this occurs the temporary restoration is often lost. There

is good evidence that following instrumentation, irrigation and the placement of an antibacterial dressing such as calcium hydroxide, the majority of infected root canals are bacteria-free. This is the optimum time to obturate the root canal system.

The root canal can be obturated when:

- There is an absence of pain and swelling.
- There is no tenderness to percussion.
- There is no patent sinus tract.
- The canal is dry.
- The canal is odour-free.
- The cleaned and shaped root canal has had a medicament placed for at least 1 week.

There has been a trend amongst specialist endodontists to undertake root canal treatment in a single visit. The rationale behind this is that delaying obturation may allow re-contamination of the root canal system. There are specific indications for such an approach, namely: the treatment of teeth with vital pulps (where microbial invasion should theoretically be minimal and multiple visits may lead to further contamination); and the situation where an immediate post crown is required.

Obturation should not be carried out immediately in the following situations:

- In teeth with apical periodontitis (radiological or symptomatic)
- Teeth with excessive exudate
- Teeth with purulent discharge
- Root canal retreatment
- Complex treatment such as perforation repair.

SEALERS

Root canal sealer is used to obliterate the irregularities and voids between the root canal filling material and the canal wall. A sealer improves the seal of the root canal filling and should be antibacterial. The material should ideally have the capability of binding to the core material and bonding to the dentine of the root canal wall. It should fill the voids that occur between the walls of the canal and the core material, and fill lateral canals and anastomoses that may not be filled by gutta percha. In cold lateral condensation sealer fills the spaces between cones of gutta percha. The sealer also acts as a lubricant during the placement of the cones.

The ideal sealer therefore has the following properties:

* Be able to achieve a seal
* Antibacterial
* Good wetting properties
* Ability to adhere to both filling material and root canal wall
* Radiopaque
* Non-irritant and well tolerated by periapical tissues
* Insoluble in tissue fluid
* Dimensionally stable
* Easy to mix
* Good working time (especially in thermoplasticized techniques)
* Easy to remove if required (retreatment and post preparation)
* Non-staining

Unfortunately there are no materials that satisfy all the above criteria. Most sealers are absorbable when exposed to tissue fluids, and therefore the sealer becomes the weak link in providing a seal; these materials are therefore used in low volume, the majority of the root canal system being filled with the core material (gutta percha).

Types of Sealer

Sealers are mixed to a paste and set by chemical reaction. They are based on the following formulations:

* Zinc oxide and eugenol
* Calcium hydroxide
* Resin
* Glass ionomer

Radio-opacifiers are added, such as precipitated silver or bismuth salts. Binding resins such as staybelite, hydrogenated rosin ester, oleoresin and polymerized resin are added. Some sealers contain antibacterial substances such as thymol iodide and calcium hydroxide. Calcium hydroxide is unlikely to be of therapeutic benefit in eugenol-based sealers, as it is chelated by eugenol.

Zinc Oxide and Eugenol-based Sealers

Many zinc oxide and eugenol-based sealers are available, and a number are variations on Grossman's original formula. It is possible to have a sealer with extra working time (EWT) for use with heated gutta percha techniques. The eugenol in these sealers is antibacterial, but the material is porous and relatively weak when set. Zinc oxide and eugenol material extruded through the apex will produce an inflammatory reaction in the periapical tissues, and this may last some time. All zinc oxide and eugenol cements are cytotoxic, and have been shown to lead to sensitization. Pulp canal sealer (Kerr, Peterborough, UK) includes silver particles to improve the radiopacity; this may potentially contribute to dentine staining following root canal treatment, and care should be taken when treating anterior teeth.

Examples are:

* Grossman's
* Tubliseal (Kerr)
* Roth (Roth International, Chicago, IL, USA)
* Pulp Canal Sealer (Kerr) (Fig. 7.1)

Calcium Hydroxide Sealers

These materials have been shown to have similar sealing ability to zinc oxide and eugenol preparations; however, long-term exposure to tissue fluid may possibly lead to dissolution of the material as calcium hydroxide is leached out.

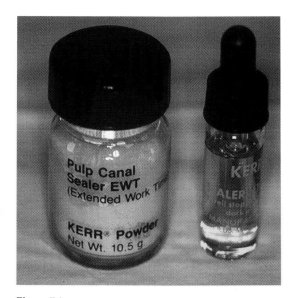

Figure 7.1

Kerr's Pulp Canal Sealer is a zinc oxide and eugenol-based sealer with extra working time. It should be mixed carefully to a relatively thick consistency.

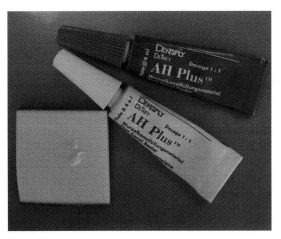

Figure 7.2

The sealer AH Plus. Equal quantities from each tube are mixed on a paper pad before use.

Example:

• Sealapex (Kerr)

Resin Sealers

The resin sealer AH26 has good sealing properties, and is adhesive and antibacterial. It is based on an epoxy resin that sets slowly when mixed with an activator. The material can initially produce a severe inflammatory reaction if present in tissue, but this subsides over a few weeks, and it is then well tolerated. These materials have the theoretical potential to be allergenic and mutagenic, and to release formaldehyde.

Examples:

• AH 26 (Dentsply, Weybridge, Surrey, UK)
• AH Plus (Dentsply) (Fig. 7.2)

Glass Ionomer Sealers

Glass ionomer cements have the ability to adhere to dentine, and for this reason would appear to be a suitable material for use as an endodontic sealer. Glass ionomer cements are cytotoxic while setting, but inflammatory reactions reduce with time. Experimentally these sealers appear to perform as well as zinc oxide and eugenol-based materials. Glass ionomer has been shown to produce a good coronal seal when used to coat the pulp floor of an endodontically treated tooth. There may be some difficulty removing set glass ionomer cement from the root canal system when carrying out root canal retreatment.

Example:

• Ketac Endo (ESPE, Seefeld, Oberlay, Germany)

ROOT FILLING MATERIALS

It is no longer considered acceptable to obturate root canals with rigid materials such as silver points. The points do not obturate the canal effectively, as they rely on large volumes of sealer to fill the voids around them. Pastes containing paraformaldehyde (e.g. N2, SPAD) are not desirable, as the material is potentially highly irritant and carcinogenic and may spread systemically throughout the body.

Gutta percha has been used to fill root canals for over a century, and remains the material of choice.

Gutta Percha

This natural rubber is the *cis* isomer of polyisoprene. Gutta percha can exist in three phases: α, β and amorphous (molten). Conventional gutta percha points exist in the β form, which transforms to the α phase on heating between 42 and 49°C; between 53 and 59°C the material enters an amorphous phase. These phase transformations are very important: heating the gutta percha during obturation results in shrinkage on cooling as the phase changes occur. Of practical importance to the dentist is the fact that heated gutta percha requires pressure to compact it as it cools, to prevent contraction gaps from developing.

Other agents are added to the gutta percha to make the points that are used in dentistry.

The typical point consists of:

	percentage	
• Gutta percha	19–22	
• Zinc oxide	59–75	—for stiffness
• Metal sulphates	1.5–17	—for radiopacity
• Waxes/resins	1–4	—for handling properties
• Colouring agent	<1	—for visual contrast

OBTURATION TECHNIQUES

There are many techniques for obturating the root canal system:

- Cold lateral condensation
- Warm lateral condensation (Fig. 7.3)
- Warm vertical condensation (Fig. 7.4)
- Thermocompaction (ultrasonic and mechanical) (Fig. 7.5)
- Injection of thermoplasticized gutta percha
- Chloropercha

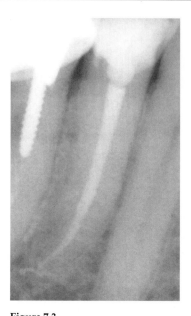

Figure 7.3

This premolar tooth has been obturated using a lateral condensation technique.

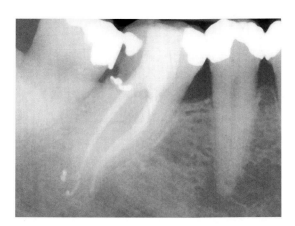

Figure 7.4

Warm vertical condensation of the root canal space. Hydraulic forces during compaction will often obturate lateral canals.

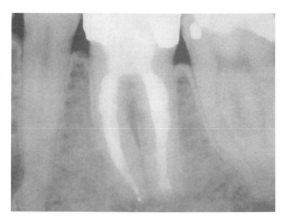

Figure 7.5

Thermoplasticized gutta percha techniques are very useful when obturating complex canal shapes. In this case the root canal system has been obturated with Obtura (Texceed Corporation, Costa Mesa, CA, USA).

Lateral Condensation

Lateral condensation is widely used, and still stands as a benchmark for new obturation techniques. Tapered cones of gutta percha are placed in the root canal and condensed with metal spreaders. The first gutta percha cone is known as the master cone, and this corresponds in size to the ISO size of the master apical file. Hand or finger spreaders can be used to condense the gutta percha points. Less force can be applied to the walls of the root canal using a finger spreader, and for this reason they are safer (Fig. 7.6). When using greater tapered root canal instruments it is possible to produce a relatively predictable taper to the prepared root canal. A master point can then be selected that not only corresponds to the master apical size but also to the taper. By using such a cone the bulk of the root canal space is obturated immediately, reducing the number of accessory cones that will be required to fill the canal completely. Traditional cold lateral condensation is particularly wasteful of gutta percha cones, and the canal orifices can be completely obliterated with a 'mushroom' of accessory point bulging from the access cavity! (Figs. 7.7–7.10).

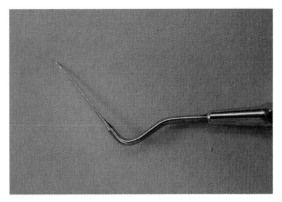

Figure 7.6

The tip of a hand spreader.

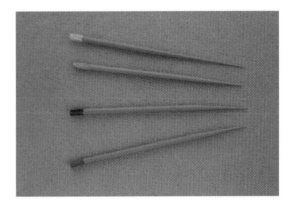

Figure 7.7

Gutta percha manufactured to correspond to the Greater Taper files (Dentsply), in tapers 0.06, 0.08, 0.10, 0.12.

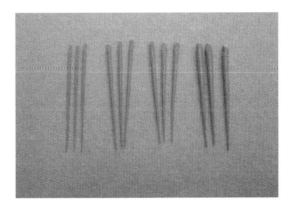

Figure 7.8

Accessory gutta percha points in sizes A–D.

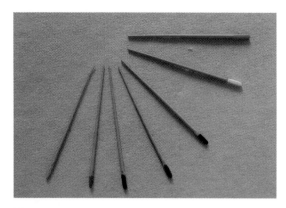

Figure 7.9

Gutta percha points in ISO sizes.

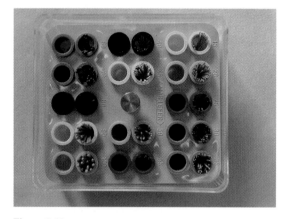

Figure 7.10

The ISO points are manufactured in a wide range of sizes that correspond to the hand files.

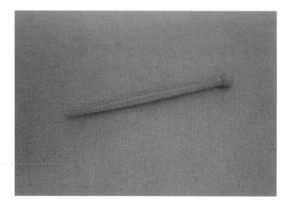

Figure 7.11

A customized cone has been rolled on a glass slab.

The Technique

Cone Fitting

A standardized gutta percha point of the same size as the master apical file or a non-standardized gutta percha point that corresponds to the taper of the completed root canal preparation is selected. Non-standard taper cones usually need to be trimmed at their tip to correspond to the diameter of the apical preparation.

The point is then inserted into the canal, and should exhibit 'tug-back' at a point 0.5–1.0 mm short of the working length.

A finger spreader when inserted on the outer curve of the canal wall alongside the point will drive it to the full working length.

Custom-fitting a Gutta Percha Cone

Occasionally the apical size of the prepared root canal may be larger than a standardized cone. In this case a customized gutta percha cone will need to be formed. The chloroform dip technique is useful in this situation.

- The cone is fitted so that tug-back is felt just short of the working length. Sometimes it is necessary to prefabricate the cone by rolling a large gutta percha point between two glass slabs, or alternatively, by blending several smaller points together in the same manner (Fig. 7.11).
- Dip the tip of the gutta percha point in solvent (e.g. chloroform) (Fig. 7.12).
- Place the cone immediately into the prepared root canal to the working length (Fig. 7.13).
- On removal the tip will have adapted to irregularities at the apical end of the root canal (Fig. 7.14).
- A thin coating of sealer is applied to the gutta percha, and the cone is refitted into the root canal.
- During lateral condensation excessive forces should be avoided to prevent displacing the master cone apically.

Lateral Condensation

After selection of a suitable point, root canal sealer is mixed and inserted in the canal. All walls should be coated evenly with a thin layer, and this can be achieved with a paper point, a hand file or an endosonic file

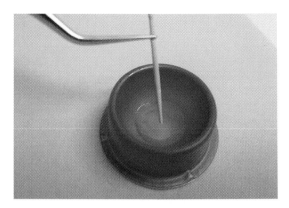

Figure 7.12

The tip is dipped in chloroform.

(Fig. 7.15). The master cone is then dipped in sealer and inserted into the canal. It is condensed into place with the finger spreader placed between it and the outer wall of the curved canal wall. The spreader is pushed and rotated back and forth 45°. The size of spreader will depend on the taper of the preparation and the degree of curvature of the canal (Fig. 7.16). The tip of the instrument should pass to within a few millimetres of the working length at the start of compaction (Fig. 7.17). Following lateral compaction the instrument is withdrawn slowly.

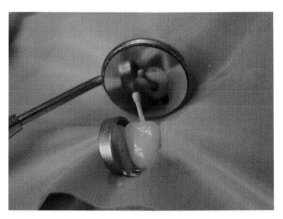

Figure 7.13

The cone is immediately seated to working length.

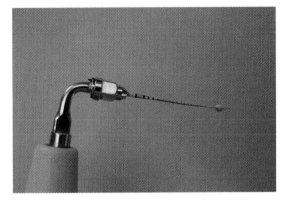

Figure 7.15

Endosonics is highly effective for coating the walls of the root canal with sealer.

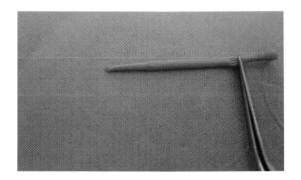

Figure 7.14

The tip has adapted to irregularities within the apical end of the root canal.

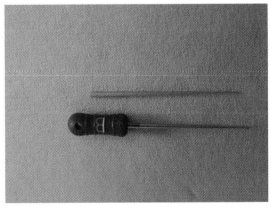

Figure 7.16

A size B finger spreader and equivalent accessory point.

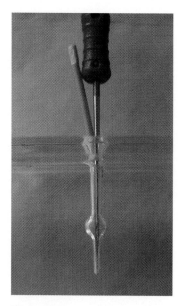

Figure 7.17

The spreader should be inserted to within a few millimetres of the working length at the start of condensation (shown here in a transparent block).

An accessory point of similar size to the spreader is chosen and placed into the vacated space. The spreader is again replaced between the gutta percha and the outer wall of the curved canal, and the procedure is repeated until the canal is filled. As condensation progresses the spreader will penetrate less far.

Removal of Excess Gutta Percha
The gutta percha points protruding into the pulp chamber can be removed with a heated instrument, such as an old excavator. The top of the root filling can be condensed vertically with a cold plugger. The root canal filling should be finished flush with the orifice. Finally, a radiograph should be taken to verify that the filling is properly placed and adequately condensed without voids.

Warm Lateral Condensation

In this technique heat is used to thermoplasticize the gutta percha and compact points. With any technique using heat it is important to apply pressure to the gutta percha during cooling to counteract the shrinkage that occurs as the filling material undergoes phase changes on cooling.

By applying heat to the gutta percha the forces required for compaction are reduced. It is also possible to adapt the thermoplasticized material to the irregularities within the canal.

The Technique

Cone Fitting
The gutta percha points used in heated techniques are designed to thermoplasticize easily, and their containers sometimes bear the inscription 'suitable for the Schilder technique'.

A non-standardized gutta percha point that corresponds to the taper of the completed root canal preparation is selected. The tip of the cone is trimmed to correspond to the diameter of the apical preparation. The point when inserted into the canal should exhibit 'tug-back' at a point 0.5–1.0 mm short of the working length.

Warm Lateral Condensation (Fig. 7.18)
After selection of a suitable point, root canal sealer is mixed and inserted in the canal as previously. The master cone is then dipped in sealer and inserted into the canal. It is condensed into place with the finger spreader placed between it and the outer curve of the canal wall. The spreader is pushed and rotated back and forth 45°. The size of spreader will depend on the taper of the preparation and the degree of curvature of the canal. The tip of the instrument should pass to within a few millimetres of the working length at the start of compaction. Following lateral compaction the instrument is withdrawn slowly.

Application of Heat
Heat can be applied to the gutta percha using:

1. A heat carrier
2. An electrically heated tip (e.g. Touch and Heat, or System B: both Analytic Endodontics, Redmond, WA, USA) (Fig. 7.19)
3. An ultrasonic tip (Figs. 7.20, 7.21)

Heat carriers are held in a Bunsen flame or a

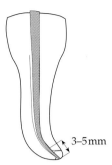

A cone is selected that corresponds to the apical dimension and taper of the prepared root canal. It is fitted to the working length with tug-back.

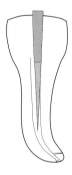

A light coating of sealer is placed on to the walls of the root canal using a hand file, endosonic file or gutta percha point.

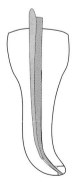

A cold finger spreader is inserted alongside the master cone and gentle lateral condensation is applied. A heated spreader is then placed in the space and used to adapt the gutta percha whilst it is thermoplasticized. Spreaders should be removed from the canal when they are cold to avoid displacing the gutta percha. Pressure should be applied to counteract the shrinkage that occurs during cooling.

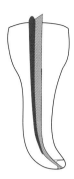

An accessory cone is coated in sealer and inserted into the space created by the spreaders. The sequence for lateral condensation is the same as before: cold finger spreader first followed by the heated spreader. Gentle lateral forces are used to adapt the cones while cooling.

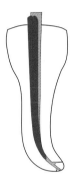

The process is repeated with more accessory cones.

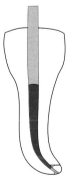

The gutta percha cones are cut off level with the pulp floor using an electric heater tip or hot instrument. Vertical pressure is applied with a cold plugger for several seconds.

Figure 7.18

Warm lateral condensation.

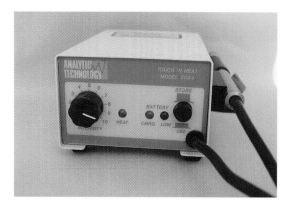

Figure 7.19

The touch and heat electric heater.

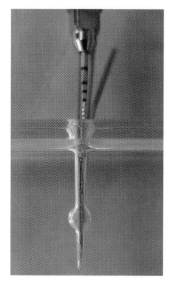

Figure 7.20

An endosonic tip can be used to heat the gutta percha.

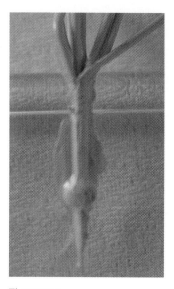

Figure 7.21

The ultrasonic thermoplasticized gutta percha is compacted into all the canal irregularities of the transparent plastic block.

- Place heated spreader into canal and laterally condense until cool.
- Remove the spreader cold (thereby allowing for contraction and reducing the risk of removing the gutta percha with the instrument).
- Insert accessory cone and sealer.
- Repeat process until the canal is filled.

Removal of Excess Gutta Percha
The gutta percha points protruding into the pulp chamber can be removed as described previously.

salt bead sterilizer and carried to the root canal for use. Electrically heated tips offer more control, allowing the precise delivery of heat where it is required at the press of a button. Some clinicians use ultrasonically energized spreader tips to achieve thermal condensation.

The sequence of heat application is as follows:

- Make space for heated instrument with a cold spreader.

Vertical Compaction of Gutta Percha (Fig. 7.22)

Vertical condensation techniques involve the compaction of heated gutta percha in an apical direction using a variety of methods to deliver the heat.

Excessive flow of the obturating material apically must be resisted to avoid extrusion; this is ensured by creating a tapered preparation. The

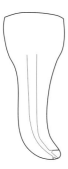

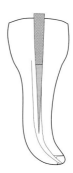

The completed preparation should be tapered. As the diameter decreases the resistance to flow increases. Keeping the apical preparation as small as practical prevents extrusion of filling material.

A light coating of sealer is placed on the walls of the canal, using a hand file, and onto the gutta percha point.

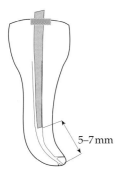

5–7 mm

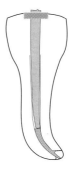

The System B tip is pre-measured. It should fit passively 5–7 mm from the working length. A rubber stop is used to mark the length against a reference point.

The down pack

- The cone is cut off level with the pulp floor using the system B tip.
- Light pressure is applied with a cold Machtou plugger (Maillefer, Bellaigues, Switzerland).
- The activated System B tip is plunged apically into the gutta percha until the stop is 2–3 mm short of the reference point.
- The wave of compaction is continued without heat until the rubber stop is at the reference point.
- Apical pressure is applied for 10 seconds as the gutta percha cools.
- A short burst of heat is applied and the System B tip is removed.
- A cold plugger is used to compact the apical segment of gutta percha.

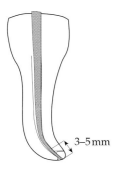

3–5 mm

A tapered cone is selected that corresponds to the completed preparation. If the tip of the gutta percha point is too small then it can be trimmed with scissors. 'Tug-back' should be felt when the fit is correct.

Figure 7.22

Vertical compaction: System B..

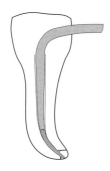

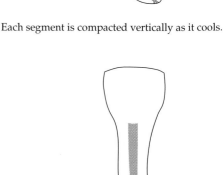

The backfill

- The coronal portion of the canal is empty. It can be obturated using small segments of heated gutta percha.
- When using the Obtura system, the tip should be inserted gently into the apical mass of gutta percha before injecting. Light apical pressure should be maintained as the gutta percha is injected into the root canal.
- Alternatively, small segments of a gutta percha point can be placed in the canal, heated with the System B tip and compacted using cold Machtou pluggers.

Figure 7.22 (contd)

Each segment is compacted vertically as it cools.

The canal is filled to the level of the pulp floor.

smallest diameter is apical and the greatest coronal; resistance to flow increases as the diameter of the preparation decreases. The gutta percha is heated and then condensed with each plugger in an apical direction. The maximum cross-section of gutta percha should be captured by each plugger without binding on the canal walls. If too small a plugger is used then it either slides alongside the gutta percha or passes through it without applying apical pressure. The System B technique simplifies the original process by providing vertical compaction in a single wave in an apical direction (Fig. 7.23).

The Technique

There are three phases to the vertical compaction technique

- Cone fit
- Down pack
- Back fill

The Cone Fit

Gutta percha points used in vertical compaction techniques must thermoplasticize easily.

A non-standardized gutta percha point that corresponds to the taper of the completed root canal preparation is selected. The tip of the cone is trimmed to correspond to the diameter of the apical preparation. The point when inserted into the canal should exhibit 'tug-back' 0.5–1.0 mm short of the working length (Fig. 7.24).

Measuring the Plugger

A plugger should be selected for the system B electric heater that fits to within 5–7 mm of the working length, without binding excessively on the canal walls.

This point is marked with a rubber stop (Fig. 7.25).

A hand plugger (Schilder or Machtou plug-

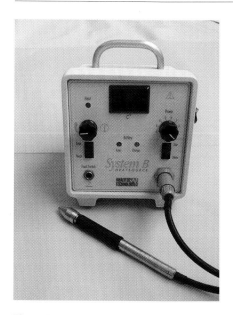

Figure 7.23

The system B unit.

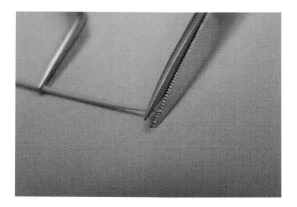

Figure 7.24

If the tip of the gutta percha point is too small it should be trimmed to correspond to the master apical file.

ger) is also measured to the same point (Fig. 7.26).

Fitting the Cone

Sealers used in this technique must not set too quickly, and have extended working time (EWT). Sealer is applied very thinly to the walls of the canal and to the cone, which is then seated into place (Fig. 7.27).

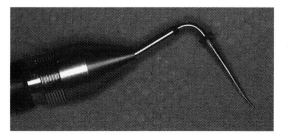

Figure 7.25

The System B plugger has been marked with a rubber stop. Touching the spring on the handle causes the tip to heat up instantly.

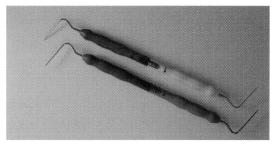

Figure 7.26

Machtou pluggers are used to compact the gutta percha following heating.

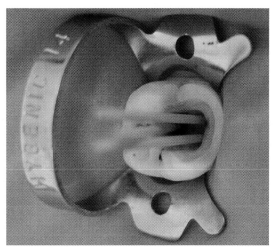

Figure 7.27

In this case all the gutta percha cones have been fitted before compaction. Gutta percha will often flow between the mesial canals during compaction, and may prevent correct insertion of a second master cone if the canals are obturated individually.

The Down Pack

The cone is cut off at the level of the pulp floor using the System B tip and then gentle force is applied with a cold plugger. The System B tip is then held at the canal orifice. The heater is activated and the tip is pushed into the mass of gutta percha in an apical direction until the stop is 3 mm short of the desired length. The finger is then removed from the heater switch and the plugger is pushed the final distance without applying heat. Once at the working length the tip is held in place for 10 seconds (to counteract the shrinkage that will occur as the gutta percha cools). A quick pulse of heat is applied and the tip is removed. (Gutta percha may well be seen coating the plugger.) The cold hand plugger is immediately inserted into the canal to apply apical pressure for a further 20 seconds.

The Backfill

The empty coronal portion of the root canal is easily obturated using thermoplasticized gutta percha delivered by a suitable system (e.g. Obtura or heated sections of gutta percha cone: Fig. 7.28). Several aliquots of gutta percha are inserted into the canal and plugged individually using cold hand pluggers to reduce the cooling shrinkage. The obturating material is then finished level with the pulp floor (Fig. 7.29).

TROUBLESHOOTING OBTURATION TECHNIQUES

Master Cone Will Not Fit to Length

- Dentine chips packed into the apical extent of the root canal preparation will lead to a decrease in working length, and consequently the master cone will appear to be short. This can be avoided by using copious amounts of irrigant during preparation. (See section on preparation.)
- A ledge in the root canal wall can prevent correct placement of the cone. If the cone hits an obstruction during placement then the end may appear crinkled (Fig. 7.30). It may be possible to remove or smooth a ledge by refining the preparation with a greater taper instrument.

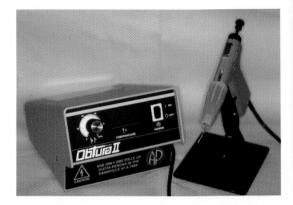

Figure 7.28

The Obtura II system.

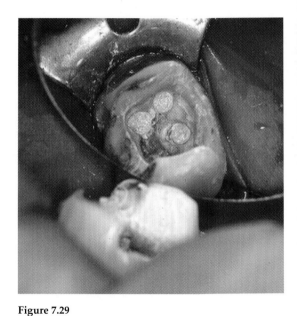

Figure 7.29

Following backfilling the gutta percha is condensed level with the pulp floor.

- If the canal is insufficiently tapered, the master cone may not fit correctly because it is binding against the canal walls coronally or in the mid-third. The completed root canal preparation should follow a gradual taper along its entire length. Further preparation may be required with Gates-Glidden burs, orifice shapers or a greater taper instrument.

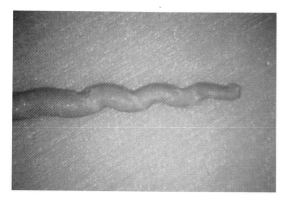

Figure 7.30

Crinkling of the gutta percha point is often caused by the tip hitting an obstruction.

- Check the size and taper of the master cone. Gutta percha cones are not perfectly standardized. Another cone from the same box may fit.

Inability to Place the Spreader/Plugger to Length

- If the root canal preparation is inadequately tapered the spreader or plugger may bind in the coronal or mid-third. In this case there will not be enough room to place the instrument to the desired length. The preparation should be refined with Gates-Glidden burs, orifice shapers, or a greater taper instrument.
- It is important to select the correct size of spreader/plugger. A System B tip should fit passively to within 5–7 mm of the working length. For example, an FM tip should fit most 0.08 tapered preparations.
- Spreaders and System B pluggers can be precurved to conform to the curved canal shapes if they are binding in a curved canal.

Removing Cones during Condensing

- If a cone has poor tug-back because it does not fit correctly, then it is more likely to be removed during condensation.
- Too much sealer acts as a lubricant; only a light coating is required.
- Sticky deposits of sealer on the spreader may dislodge the gutta percha cones. Instruments must be wiped clean after each use.
- Spreaders that have damaged tips or bent shanks should be discarded.
- Sufficient space should be made during lateral condensation to compact the gutta percha cones before attempting to remove the spreader.
- When using an electrically activated spreader to heat the gutta percha during warm lateral condensation the tip should be allowed to cool before removing it from the root canal. Removing the tip while it is hot will result in gutta percha being removed from the canal. Continue laterally condensing as the tip cools, thereby creating space before removal.

Voids in the Obturating Material

- Poor penetration of a finger spreader will prevent accessory cones from fitting correctly. Voids will be created between the cones. A smaller spreader may be required.
- When using a vertical compaction technique, a void may appear between the downpack and backfill if the Obtura tip is not placed deep enough into the canal. The tip should be inserted until it just sinks into the apical mass of gutta percha, before injecting thermoplasticized gutta percha.
- It is tempting to withdraw the Obtura tip prematurely during backfilling as gutta percha is delivered, resulting in a void. Slight apical pressure must be applied as gutta percha is extruded from the Obtura tip. Pressure created within the root canal will gently force the needle back out of the canal.

FURTHER READING

Buchanan LS (1996). The continuous wave of obturation technique: 'centered' condensation of warm gutta percha in 12 seconds. *Dentistry Today* **15(1):** 60–62, 64–67.

Liewehr F, Kulild JC, Primack PD (1993). Improved density of gutta-percha after warm lateral condensation. *Journal of Endodontics* **19:** 489–491.

Schilder H (1967). Filling root canals in three dimensions. *Dental Clinics of North America* **11:** 723–744.

8 ROOT CANAL RETREATMENT

CONTENTS • Introduction • Why? • When? • How? • Post Removal • Ledges • Perforations • Preparation of Root Canals • Further Reading

INTRODUCTION

When root canal treatment fails there are three possible ways of dealing with the problem:

- Root canal retreatment
- Root end surgery
- Extraction.

Root Canal Retreatment

The existing root filling is removed and the infected root canal is disinfected using irrigants and medicaments. This is often the preferred treatment modality for a failed root filling. Root canal retreatment can be complicated since restorations may need to be dismantled in order to gain access to the canal system. The tooth should be assessed for restorability before this prolonged and often expensive treatment is started. If the tooth is unrestorable then it may be better to extract it and provide an alternative replacement.

Root-End Surgery

Placing a root-end filling in a tooth with an infected root canal will undoubtedly lead to failure. Surgery is normally reserved for cases in which root canal treatment or retreatment has been unsuccessful. Often a surgical approach is difficult and may be beyond the expertise of the operator.

Extraction

Removing the tooth may be the best option if the tooth is unrestorable or the prognosis for root canal retreatment is poor. It is not possible to save every tooth.

WHY?

It has been shown that high success rates can be achieved for root canal retreatment, especially when failure of the existing root treatment was due to technical inadequacy.

Root canal retreatment encompasses the problems encountered with routine root canal treatment: invariably an infected root canal system; fine canals, fins, tight curves and other complex anatomy combined with iatrogenic difficulties; and existing root filling materials, broken instruments, ledges and perforations. Retreatment is therefore more demanding than primary root canal treatment. Patients are becoming more reluctant to have teeth extracted, and difficult root canal retreatment may require specialist equipment and expertise. Referral to an endodontist should be offered to patients when the technical difficulties exceed the practitioner's capabilities.

WHEN?

Root canal retreatment may be considered when:

- Persistent pain or symptoms develop in a tooth that has received root canal treatment
- The existing root treatment is deficient technically
- There have been procedural errors
- A new coronal restoration (such as a crown) is planned on a tooth with a technically deficient root canal filling or in the presence of nonresolving periapical radiolucencies.

HOW?

Retreatment

Some of the retreatment problems faced in practice are:

- Paste and cement root filling materials
- Silver points
- Fractured instruments
- Post removal
- Ledges
- Perforations.

Illumination and Magnification

Good illumination is essential for predictable root canal treatment. As retreatment cases are generally more demanding than previously untreated cases, it is almost impossible, while working at the base of a dark access cavity using tactile sense alone, to locate missed root canals, separated instruments or filling material lodged in the complex anatomy. Magnification can best be achieved with loupes that have an additional headlamp or with a surgi-

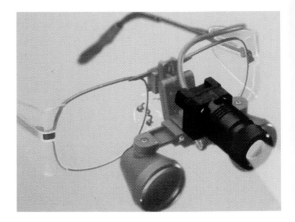

Figure 8.1

Loupes with illumination in the direction of sight.

cal microscope. Loupes offer magnification in the range ×2.5 to ×4, which is ideal for endodontics and routine dentistry. The advantage of such a system over using an operating light is that the light source is much brighter and is directed in the line of sight (Fig. 8.1). Microscopes offer excellent illumination and very high magnification but are considerably more expensive. Most endodontic specialists use microscopes routinely.

Paste and Cement Root Filling Materials

Paste and cement root filling materials include calcium hydroxide-based pastes, zinc oxide and eugenol cements, and Endomethazone (Septodent, Deprow, Maidstone, Kent, UK). Pastes are not recommended as permanent root canal filling materials. During the removal of pastes, extrusion of material into the periodontal space and excessive damage to the root canal walls must be prevented.

Removing Paste from the Pulp Chamber

Nonsetting materials can be effectively removed from the pulp chamber using:

- An ultrasonic scaler tip (Fig. 8.2)
- An excavator
- Irrigant in a syringe.

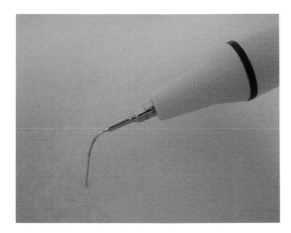

Figure 8.2

An ultrasonic scaler tip can be used to remove material from the pulp chamber.

The irrigant flow on the ultrasonic scaler should be set at maximum. Acoustic micro-streaming and cavitation will dislodge paste material and wash it away.

Removing Paste from Root Canals

Paste can be removed from root canals:

- During coronal flaring
- With endosonics
- With hand irrigation.

If a root canal has been underprepared, coronal flaring will remove significant amounts of material early in the preparation sequence. Coronal flaring is normally carried out at the start of modern preparation techniques, either with a combination of files and Gates-Glidden burs or with nickel–titanium rotary instruments.

Paste materials in the apical regions of canal systems can be removed using endosonics. Although cavitation is unlikely to occur within the confines of a canal system, acoustic microstreaming and a high volume of irrigant will help remove paste from the canals.

Set Cements

Set cements are extremely difficult to remove from the root canal system and require mechanical removal using:

- Ultrasonic scaler tip
- Specialist ultrasonic tips (such as CT and CPR) (Fig. 8.3)
- An endosonic tip with shortened file
- Round burs
- Solvents.

Material can be removed in a controlled manner using a piezoelectric ultrasonic handpiece with a scaler tip or specialist CT and CPR tips. Ultrasonic vibration breaks up the cement and is preferably used with irrigant.

Removing material from the root canal with a round bur should really be a method of last resort, unless it is possible to see directly where the bur is cutting, since there is a high risk of perforation. As swan neck burs have a flexible shaft, there is a tendency to wander sideways while cutting. This could result in lateral perforation. The need for illumination and magnification cannot be overemphasized.

Gutta Percha Removal

The Single Cone

Single cone gutta percha root fillings can usually be removed using:

- A Hedstroem file
- Tweezers

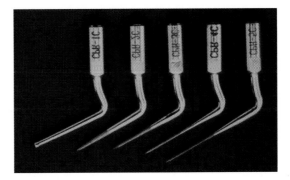

Figure 8.3

The CPR set of ultrasonic tips: 1C is for vibrating posts, 2C and 3C are for work on the pulp floor, and 4C and 5C are for use within the confines of root canal.

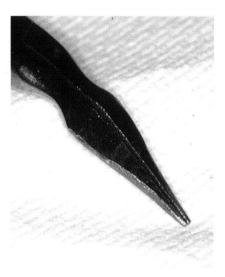

Figure 8.4

These Stieglitz forceps have been modified to make the beak thinner.

- Stieglitz forceps (Fig. 8.4)
- Endosonics.

Hedstroem files are weakest in a rotary direction and therefore the largest Hedstroem file that will fit alongside the cone should be used to help reduce the risk of file fracture. The file is gently screwed into the canal alongside the gutta percha cone until resistance is met. At this point, the instrument is withdrawn from the canal, along with the gutta percha cone. Endosonics may loosen cement around a single cone, thereby aiding removal. Cones can be gripped with tweezers or Stieglitz forceps for removal.

Condensed Gutta Percha

Condensed gutta percha can be removed using a combination of:

- Heat
- Gates-Glidden burs
- Nickel–titanium rotary instruments
- Hand instruments such as Hedstroem files
- Solvents.

Heat

Heat is a useful means of removing gutta percha from the coronal portion of a root canal. A System B tip (Analytic Endodontics; Redmond, WA, USA) or heated plugger can be used.

Gates-Glidden Burs, Rotary Instruments and Hedstroem Files

When a root filling is well compacted, as much gutta percha as possible should be removed from the root canal system before solvent is used. Gates-Glidden burs are extremely efficient for removing gutta percha from the coronal parts of the root canal. They need to be rotated in a slow handpiece at reasonable speed, generating frictional heat that will aid gutta percha removal.

Rotary nickel–titanium instruments can also be used to remove gutta percha; the orifice openers are particularly effective and need to be rotated at 600 rpm.

A Hedstroem file is then used to remove any free cones and further fragments of gutta percha. Finally, a few drops of solvent (e.g. chloroform) are placed in the canal. Files are used to remove the bulk of dissolved gutta percha. The file is rotated into the mass of gutta percha and withdrawn; it is then wiped clean on a gauze square and the process is repeated. Finally, a few more drops of chloroform are placed in the root canal and paper points are used to wick any remaining dissolved gutta percha. When the paper points are clean on removal, the root canal system should be completely devoid of gutta percha filling material (Figs. 8.5–8.7).

Solvents for Gutta Percha

Solvents include chloroform, xylene, rectified turpentine, methyl chloroform and eucalyptus oil. There has been some concern expressed in the literature about the carcinogenic potential of chloroform. It should only be used in small amounts and must be contained within the root canal system. Rectified turpentine is a useful alternative. Eucalyptus oil must be heated in order to be effective. Glass or polypropylene syringes should be

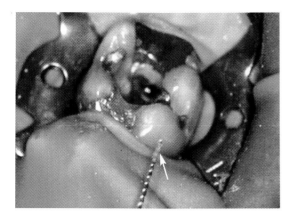

Figure 8.5

Dissolved gutta percha is being removed on the tip of a Hedstroem file (arrow).

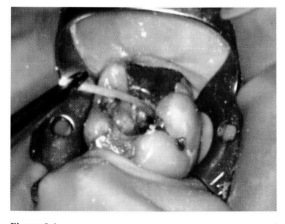

Figure 8.6

Paper points are used to wick the remaining dissolved gutta percha from the root canals.

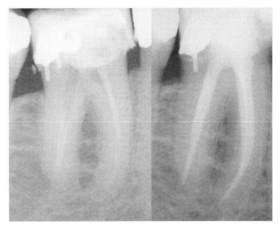

Figure 8.7

A typical gutta percha retreatment case. The existing root filling was removed using Gates-Glidden burs and Hedstroem files followed by chloroform wicking. The second canal in the mesial root was located. Following this all the canals were thoroughly disinfected before being filled with gutta percha and sealer.

Thermafil

A Thermafil obturator (Dentsply, Weybridge, Surrey, UK) consists of a carrier coated with gutta percha; it is used in conjunction with sealer to obturate the root canal system. When removing Thermafil, it is easier to remove the carrier first and then remove the gutta percha. The modern carriers have a V-shaped notch along one side, beside which a Hedstroem file can be inserted. When the file is withdrawn, the carrier is usually removed. The remaining gutta percha can be removed as previously described. Plastic carriers are also soluble in some of the solvents used to remove gutta percha (such as chloroform).

used to dispense small amounts of these solvents, since they are not dissolved. Using chloroform too early in treatment leaves a messy layer of dissolved gutta percha coating the root canals and pulp floor, which can then be difficult to remove. If most of the gutta percha has been removed mechanically, then a minimal amount of chloroform is required to dissolve the remaining filling material completely.

Silver Points and Fractured Instruments

The position of the silver point within the root canal will dictate the degree of difficulty in removal:

- Coronal position – easy
- Middle position – intermediate
- Apical position – difficult.

Coronal Position

If the coronal end of the silver point extends into the pulp chamber, then it should be preserved. Cement can be removed carefully from around the point using a Piezon ultrasonic unit (EMS: Forestgate, Dallas, TX, USA) and CT4 tip or scaler tip. Great care must be taken not to sever the point and damage the coronal end. The point is withdrawn using Stieglitz forceps or small-ended artery forceps (Figs. 8.8–8.10).

If a point has fractured within the canal or has been cut off at the level of the pulp chamber floor, then removal is more difficult. Fractured instruments present a similar problem.

In the coronal portion of the root canal, a trough can be created around the object using specialist ultrasonic tips (such as CT4 or UT). These are used to remove dentine and they can be used dry or with irrigant. Gently working a Hedstroem file between the point and the canal wall may allow it to be removed. An endosonic file gently inserted alongside a point may loosen cement and dislodge it.

Apical Position

Removing silver points from the apical third is extremely difficult. Two techniques can be

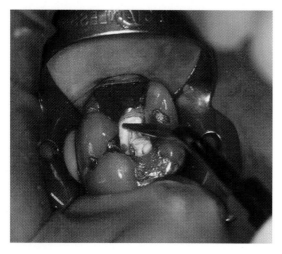

Figure 8.8

The core around the heads of the silver points being dismantled using a CT4 ultrasonic tip.

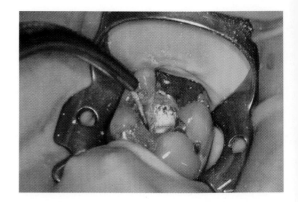

Figure 8.9

A silver point being withdrawn using fine artery forceps.

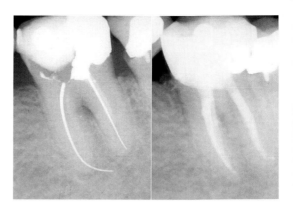

Figure 8.10

With care it is possible to remove a silver point even when it is broken off at the level of the pulp floor and overextended.

used in this region of the root canal system:

- Braiding
- Cancellier.

Braiding is a technique that can be used to remove pieces of fractured instrument or silver point from deeper in the root canal system. Although originally described using ISO size 15 files, the largest size possible should be used to help reduce the risk of file fracture. The first Hedstroem file is gently screwed into the canal alongside the object, and two further Hedstroem files are then gently inserted. These files are then wound around each other and withdrawn together (Figs. 8.11 and 8.12). The object should be gripped by the files and removed.

A Cancellier is effectively a hollow tube that can be inserted over a fractured instrument within the root canal. A small drop of cyanoacrylate adhesive is used to bond the two and then the instrument is withdrawn (Fig. 8.13).

Middle Position

The basic principles for removing fractured instruments in the mid-third of the canal are:

1   Create space
2   Use ultrasonic vibration
3   Removal.

Space can be created using orifice openers, ultrasonics or Gates-Glidden burs. Sufficient space must be created so that ultrasonic tips can be inserted without perforating the root. A Gates-Glidden bur can be modified so that is has a flat tip; this produces a neat table of dentine around the fractured instrument and allows better access for CT tips. Under direct vision using magnification and illumination, the piece of instrument is vibrated with ultrasound; CT tips are often too thick for use within the confines of the root canal, whereas

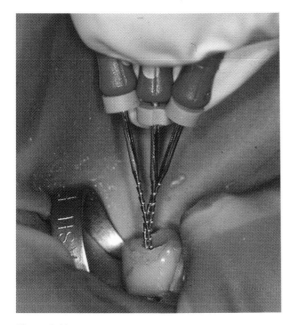

Figure 8.11

Braiding can be used to remove objects from deeper in the canal.

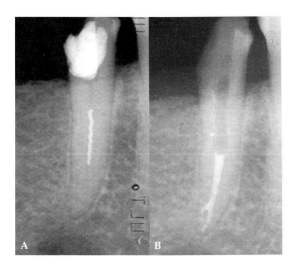

Figure 8.12

The file in this case (A) was removed using a braiding technique; the canal could then be relocated, prepared, cleaned and filled (B).

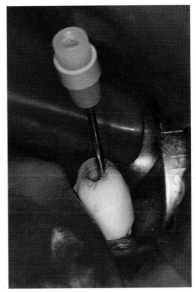

Figure 8.13

The Cancellier tube is filled with a drop of cyanoacrylate and placed over the object ready for removal.

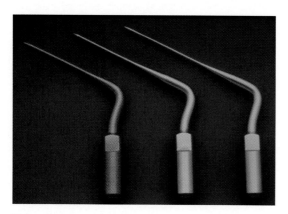

Figure 8.14

Zirconium nitride ultrasonic tips for working deep in the root canal under microscopic magnification.

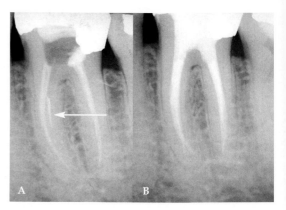

Figure 8.15

A nickel–titanium instrument fractured in the mid-third of a mesial canal (A) was removed using ultrasonics under the microscope. The canals were shaped, cleaned and filled (B).

zirconium nitride tips are longer and thinner (Fig. 8.14). Irrigant is used to wash away debris.

Once the instrument is loose then it can be removed, using braiding, a Cancellier or endosonic irrigation (Fig. 8.15).

What Happens if the Instrument is not Removable?

It is worth remembering that the pain experienced by a patient with a fractured instrument in a tooth is due to bacterial infection of the root canal space and not by the offending instrument. If the object cannot be removed, then an attempt should be made to bypass it, allowing penetration of irrigants beyond and around the fragment to disinfect the root canal. Gently working a small file alongside the fractured instrument using ethylene diamine tetra-acetic acid (EDTA) to soften dentine may create enough space to bypass fragment. If this is not possible, the root canal should be cleaned thoroughly and obturated to the level of the blockage.

POST REMOVAL

Screw Posts

A post with a screwhead, such as a Dentatus (Tricare, Bradford, UK) or Radix (Maillefer,

Ballaigues, Switzerland) anchor, can usually be removed by cutting away any adherent core material and using a wrench to unscrew it (Fig. 8.16). Placing an ultrasonic scaler tip on the post will loosen it, and it may even start to unscrew. Posts that are fractured beneath the pulp floor can be removed with either ultrasound or the Masserann kit. Special long-necked ISO 006 burs are available to cut a trough around posts that are fractured at the level of the root face, but extreme caution should be taken to avoid perforation (Fig. 8.17).

The Masserann Kit

The Masserann kit is designed for the removal of objects from the root canal. It consists of a range of trephine drills and a Masserann extractor (Fig. 8.18). The trephine is used to create a space around an object. The extractor tube is then inserted over the fractured instrument or silver point, which is then gripped by screwing in a rod. The hole required to fit the Masserann extractor is relatively large and significant amounts of dentine are removed. It should therefore only be used in the coronal third of the canal, where access is relatively straight, to avoid perfora-

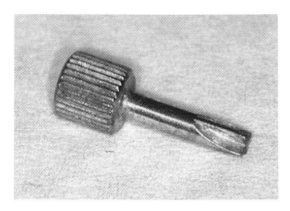

Figure 8.16

The Dentatus wrench.

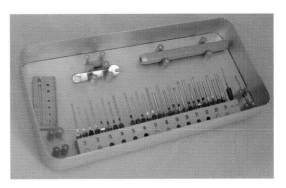

Figure 8.18

The Masserann kit.

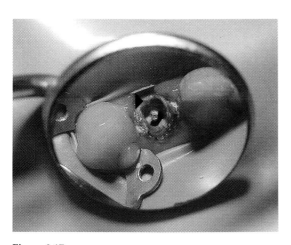

Figure 8.17

An attempt has been made to remove the post with a bur. Excessive dentine has been removed (arrow) resulting in a weakened, unrestorable tooth.

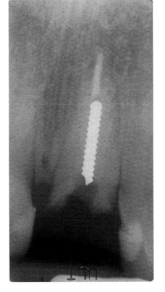

Figure 8.19

A radiograph of a fractured post that was removed using the Masserann kit and ultrasonics.

tion. The trephines are fragile and can be easily blunted. The cutting tips should be checked before use and can be sharpened carefully with a carborundum disc.

Larger objects can be removed using the Masserann trephines, which are rotated by hand or in a handpiece, cutting in an anti-clockwise direction. Once luting cement has been removed from around the object, the next smallest trephine can be used to grip it for removal (Figs. 8.19–8.23).

Cast Posts

An ultrasonic scaler tip or Piezon ultrasonic tips (Fig. 8.24) can be used for vibrating a post to break up the cement lute surrounding it. A notch can be cut in the post for placement of an ultrasonic tip, which is oscillated against the post in a vertical direction.

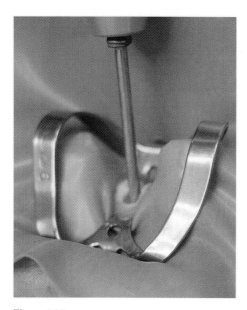

Figure 8.20

Space is made around the tip of the post using a Masserann trephine.

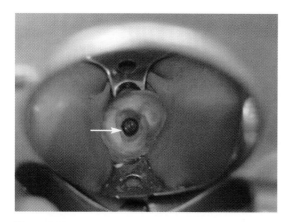

Figure 8.21

The minimal removal of dentine can be seen (arrow).

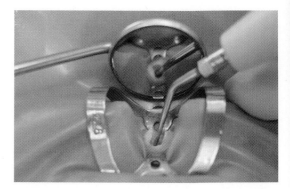

Figure 8.22

Ultrasonics are used to vibrate the post.

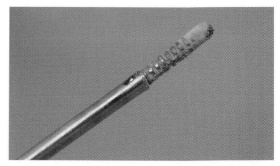

Figure 8.23

The post was then removed with a further trephine.

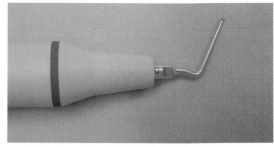

Figure 8.24

The 1CPR tip for vibrating posts ultrasonically.

Post Pullers

There are several types of post puller:

- Eggler (Fig. 8.25)
- Ruddle (Fig. 8.26)
- Gonon.

They are all used in a similar fashion; one part grips the post while the other pushes against the root face. Post pullers can be cumbersome and care should be taken not to place torsional forces on the root, since this may cause root fracture.

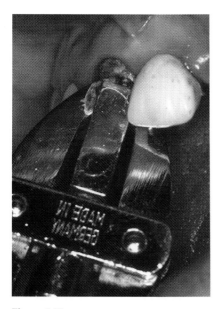

Figure 8.25

Post pullers require adequate space for use; in this case a post is being removed from a lateral incisor.

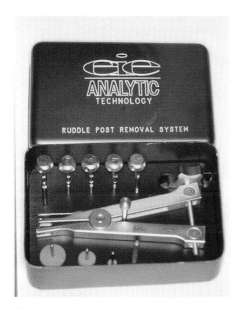

Figure 8.26

The Ruddle post removing kit. A trephine is screwed onto the post. As the jaws of the post puller open the post is withdrawn from the canal.

LEDGES

Ledges are created during root canal treatment as a result of the incorrect use of root canal instruments. A small file (such as ISO size 006 or 008) with a tight curve in the tip will sometimes allow negotiation beyond a ledge when used with a watch-winding action. A lubricant may be helpful. Once the ledge has been bypassed, the file is worked in a filing action to attempt to smooth the ledge and allow the introduction of larger files.

PERFORATIONS

The successful repair of a perforation is dependent on three variables:

- Time since occurrence
- Size
- Location.

Successful treatment of perforations depends on the ability to seal the area and prevent infection. The earlier a perforation can be repaired the better, and the possibility of infection must be kept to a minimum.

The size of a perforation will affect the prognosis, since large perforations are more difficult to seal and are associated with more tissue destruction.

Location is probably of greatest importance. Close proximity to the gingival sulcus can lead to contamination by bacteria from the oral cavity. Perforations located below crestal bone have a better prognosis, as do those away from canal orifices (Figs. 8.27 and 8.28).

Perforations can be repaired nonsurgically using modern endodontic techniques. Direct vision is essential and treatment may require the use of a microscope. Materials used to repair perforations include Super EBA (ethoxybenzoic acid: Staident International, Staines, UK), Intermediate Restorative Material (IRM: Dentsply) and Mineral Trioxide Aggregate (MTA: Dentsply). The perforation site must be thoroughly cleaned with sodium hypochlorite before placement of the repair material. Alternatively, a calcium

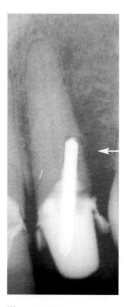

Figure 8.27

A perforation (arrow) that connects with the periodontal ligament via a pocket. The prognosis is guarded.

hydroxide dressing could be placed and the case referred for specialist treatment.

It may not be possible to achieve a successful repair of a long-term perforation, particularly if there has been periodontal breakdown.

PREPARATION OF ROOT CANALS

Following dismantling and removal of the existing root canal filling, the root canal system needs to be prepared and disinfected as with primary treatment (see Chapter 5). Sodium hypochlorite is the irrigant of choice because of its antibacterial action, and it is often used with endosonics. The bacterial ecology of retreatment cases is different from that of untreated teeth and occasionally alternative medicaments to calcium hydroxide are required (see Chapter 6).

FURTHER READING

Barbosa SV, Burkard DH, Spångberg LSW (1994). Cytotoxic effects of gutta percha solvents. *Journal of Endodontics* **20**: 6–8.

Bergenholtz G, Lekholm U, Milthon R, Heden G, Ödesjo B, Engstrom B (1979). Retreatment of endodontic fillings. *Scandinavian Journal of Dental Research* **87**: 217–224.

Hunter KR, Doblecki W, Pelleu GB Jr (1991). Halothane and eucalyptol as alternatives to chloroform for softening gutta percha. *Journal of Endodontics* **17**: 310–312.

Kaplowitz GJ (1990). Evaluation of gutta percha solvents. *Journal of Endodontics* **16**: 539–540.

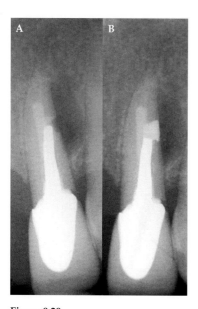

Figure 8.28

The root of this tooth has been perforated (A). The defect lies well within the alveolar bone and should have a better prognosis for healing following repair (B).

9 RESTORATION OF THE ENDODONTICALLY TREATED TOOTH

CONTENTS • Introduction • Restoration Following Root Treatment • Internal Bleaching • Simple Restoration • Extensive Restoration • Crowns • Anterior Teeth Requiring Auxiliary Retention • Posterior Teeth • Mesio-Occlusal Cavities • Conservative Cuspal Coverage Restorations • Teeth with Mesio-Occlusal-Distal Cavities • Severely Broken-Down Teeth • Temporary Crowns • Root-Filled Teeth as Abutments • Recementing a Cast Restoration or Post Crown • Further Reading

INTRODUCTION

Teeth that require endodontic treatment are often severely broken down and can be vulnerable to fracture; they often require extensive (and expensive) restoration following root canal treatment. A high fracture rate has been found in root-filled teeth that have mesial–occlusal–distal (MOD) amalgam restorations, and it is often good practice to place some form of cusp coverage restoration to prevent destructive flexure during mastication.

Sealing the Access Cavity

There is good evidence from scientific studies that the quality of coronal seal affects the prognosis of root canal treatment. It takes a relatively short time for the root-filled tooth to become reinfected if it is left exposed to the oral cavity. The root canal system must be protected from coronal leakage both during root canal treatment and after obturation.

Sealing the Access Cavity During Root Canal Treatment

After root canal preparation an antibacterial medicament is usually placed in the root canals. When the access cavity is sufficiently deep a sterile cotton wool pellet can be placed across the pulp floor and intermediate restora-

tive material (IRM: Dentsply, Weybridge, Surrey, UK) packed into the cavity. Zinc oxide and eugenol materials prevent microleakage, since the eugenol is antibacterial. Pressure should be applied to the material as it is setting to ensure good adaptation to the wall of the access cavity. The restoration can be polished with a moist cotton wool pellet (Fig. 9.1).

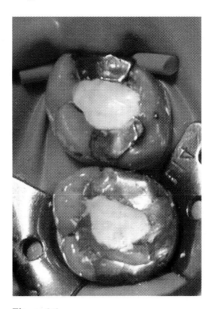

Figure 9.1

Well-adapted IRM temporaries in two maxillary molar teeth. The restorations have been burnished and polished.

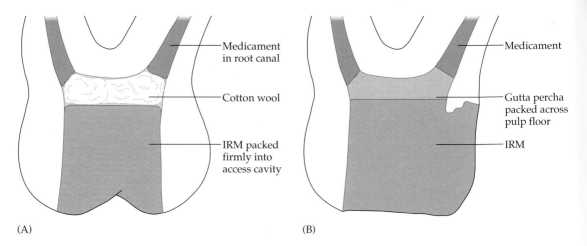

(A)   (B)

Figure 9.2

(A, B) Temporary restorations for sealing the access cavity during root canal treatment.

When there is less space, perhaps because the tooth is severely broken down or because there is decreased vertical height, a layer of thermoplasticized gutta percha such as Obtura II (Texceed Corporation, Costa Mesa, CA, USA) can be packed across the pulp floor and IRM or glass ionomer used to build up the coronal tooth substance (Fig. 9.2).

Sealing the Access Cavity Following Root Canal Treatment

The root filling material is finished at the level of the floor of the pulp chamber. A layer of IRM, glass ionomer or dentine-bonded material is placed across the pulp floor, since this approach provides a better seal than a mass of gutta percha and sealer (Fig. 9.3).

Glass ionomer materials such as Vitrebond (3M, St Paul, MN, USA) have been shown to provide a good seal and can be used in conjunction with composite or amalgam cores. An amalgam bonding agent can be used with the Nayyar core technique to provide a seal between the amalgam and dentine.

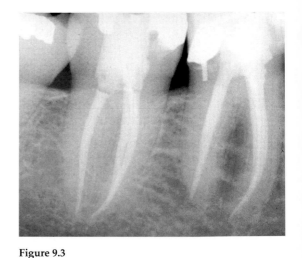

Figure 9.3

Zinc oxide and eugenol cement has been packed across the pulp floor, and it seals the entire access cavity.

RESTORATION FOLLOWING ROOT TREATMENT

Why?

Treatment Planning

The restorability of the tooth should be decided before endodontic treatment as part of an overall treatment plan. The tooth will need to be restored with an aesthetic, functional and cleansible restoration in order to protect the adjacent teeth and periodontal tissues.

Occlusal Loading

Root-filled teeth are not more brittle than unrestored teeth; however, they may be weaker as a result of unsupported or reduced tooth substance.

The likely occlusal loading can be assessed from the patient's history and a preliminary examination. Fractured restorations and teeth mobility, increased size of the muscles of mastication and faceting of occlusal contact areas may all indicate increased occlusal loading, and they all have a bearing on the treatment planning. Restoration should provide favourable distribution of any occlusal stresses within the remaining tooth substance.

Preservation of Tooth Substance

If tooth substance is conserved the remaining body of tissue will be stronger. Therefore the most conservative restoration design that complies with function, aesthetics and patient acceptance should be provided.

As a rough guideline, a full crown restoration should have a ferrule of at least 2 mm of sound dentine around the margins for optimum retention (Fig. 9.4).

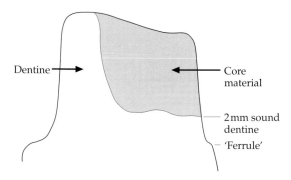

Dentine

Core material

2mm sound dentine

'Ferrule'

Figure 9.4

A full crown restoration should have margins resting on at least 2 mm of sound dentine.

Is the Tooth Restorable?

It should be decided if the tooth is restorable before endodontic treatment is carried out, and this is a primary element of the basic treatment plan. Crowns fitted on teeth that have little remaining coronal tooth tissue may require additional retention in the form of posts, pins or core material packed into the pulp space.

The patient should be made aware of the different options and their possible prognoses. Referral to a specialist may be required in some instances.

Example

The different options for restoring a fractured maxillary lateral incisor that has sheared off subgingivally in an otherwise minimally restored mouth could be:

- To do nothing – this option would probably be aesthetically unacceptable to the patient
- To construct a single tooth removable overdenture – this could be a suitable interim or temporary solution, but it would not be functionally or aesthetically acceptable as a permanent solution
- To root fill the tooth and place a post core and crown – it would be difficult to place the crown margins on sound dentine, and a post would be required to improve retention. Teeth that have been damaged in this way can be sometimes be extruded orthodontically but this is complex and the alveolar bone must be recontoured as it is extruded with the root stump. Crown lengthening may be possible to expose dentine margins, but the final result could be compromised aesthetically. The long-term prognosis of such a restoration is likely to be guarded, especially if it is not possible to finish the crown margins on sound dentine or if other cracks are present
- To extract the remaining root stump and place a cantilever bridge – an adhesive cantilever bridge would be a conservative means of restoring the space if the root were extracted. Assuming that the

occlusion was not inhibitive the prognosis and aesthetics for such a restoration should be good. Debonding is a recognized cause of failure and generally occurs between 5 and 10 years. Refixing is often appropriate. A cantilever bridge that utilizes a full coverage crown as an abutment would be much less conservative.

- To extract and replace with a single tooth implant – assuming that the placement of an osseointegrated implant was feasible then good aesthetics and a good long-term prognosis could be expected. Factors affecting the outcome of implant placement include the patient's medical history, the space available between adjacent teeth and the quality and quantity of bone. Cost may be prohibitive to the patient.

When?

Timing of Restoration

The success rates for well-executed root canal treatment should be high (80–95%) and the prognosis good. Therefore, if a patient's symptoms and signs have resolved following endodontic treatment, restoration can proceed immediately. A period of 2 weeks is usually quite sufficient, by which time the tooth should not be uncomfortable when palpated; there should also be no tenderness in the buccal sulcus or over the apex of the tooth and no evidence of a discharging sinus tract.

When teeth require a core build-up perhaps the best time to place the core is immediately after obturation. This obviates the need for a temporary restoration and provides immediate coronal seal. An amalgam core, for example in a molar tooth, can be used as an excellent interim restoration before crowning. If further endodontic intervention is required then the tooth can be easily isolated with rubber dam.

Teeth with an uncertain or guarded prognosis should be reviewed for a longer period before restoration. It is imperative, however, that the tooth should be protected from possible fracture and has good coronal seal during this interim period. Orthodontic bands can be cemented around molar teeth using zinc

phosphate cement as a temporary measure to prevent cuspal flexing. A reinforced zinc oxide and eugenol temporary restoration (e.g. IRM) will prevent microleakage, since the eugenol is antibacterial. Glass ionomer cements are also useful for sealing the access cavity.

How?

Anterior Teeth

Severely broken down anterior teeth usually require restoration for aesthetic reasons.

Teeth that need to be reviewed before definitive restoration may have to be restored with a long-term temporary. Temporary post crown restorations may not be sufficiently retentive in the long term and may not provide adequate coronal seal. In this situation it would be appropriate to fit a permanent post and core. Temporary veneer crowns can easily be fabricated over the permanent post using a blow-down splint and a syringe-mixed polymeric material (e.g. Protemp – ESPE, Seefeld, Oberlay, Germany; Luxatemp – DMG, Hamburg, Germany). If many anterior teeth are missing then an interim overdenture (Fig. 9.5) may be an alternative solution. The quality of restoration is important for endodontic success and should be addressed with both temporary and permanent restorations.

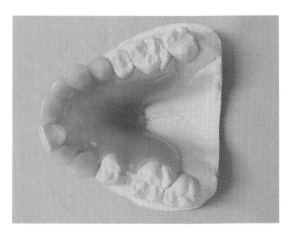

Figure 9.5

A temporary denture can sometimes be used when many anterior teeth are missing.

INTERNAL BLEACHING

Root canal-treated teeth are sometimes discoloured; however, it is not always necessary to place a crown on the tooth to improve the aesthetics. Internal (walking) bleaching is a technique that can be used after root canal treatment to lighten even severely discoloured teeth (Fig. 9.6).

How?

The root filling material is removed from the root canal to just below gingival level. Glass ionomer is then placed over the root filling. Sodium perborate powder is mixed with water to a putty consistency. This is packed into the access cavity and sealed in place with IRM. The tooth is checked 7 days later, by which time some colour change should have occurred. The process may need to be repeated two or three times to achieve the desired result. When the tooth has lightened sufficiently the access cavity can be restored with a light cured composite. The use of a shade that is lighter that the natural tooth colour can sometimes improve the appearance if the tooth is still slightly dark.

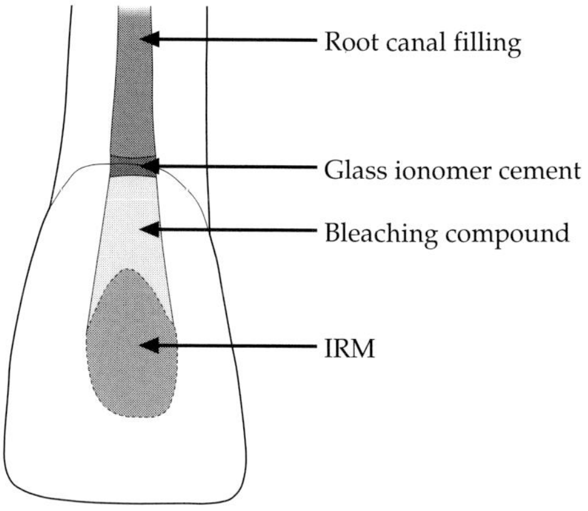

SIMPLE RESTORATION

Anterior teeth in which the majority of the coronal tooth substance is intact can normally be restored using adhesive restorative materials such as light cured composite (Figs. 9.7 and 9.8).

In moderately broken down teeth there may be sufficient tooth substance remaining to build a core using a glass ionomer cement or light cured composite to replace the missing dentine. If the buccal surface of the tooth is intact and has good aesthetics then the tooth can usually be restored with a light cured composite

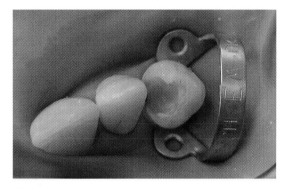

Figure 9.7

The access cavity in this canine can be restored with light cured composite. The root filling has been covered with glass ionomer.

Figure 9.6

Internal bleaching.

- Root canal filling
- Glass ionomer cement
- Bleaching compound
- IRM

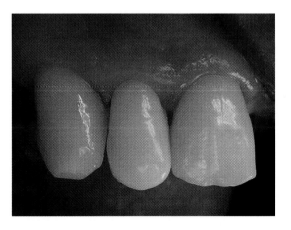

Figure 9.8

The completed composite restoration.

restoration. Glass ionomer has the advantages that it does not shrink on setting, it bonds to dentine and enamel and it leaches fluoride. If a glass ionomer and composite sandwich restoration is to be used, the tooth can be restored with glass ionomer first and then cut back and the light cured composite filling material placed at a second appointment. This allows maturation of the glass ionomer.

A total etch technique and dentine bonding agent in combination with light cured composite can be used to restore the entire cavity. Dentine is etched using an acid for approximately 10 seconds to expose collagen fibres. Primer and bond, which are often combined, are then applied to the cavity walls. This solution penetrates the layer of exposed collagen fibres to give an interface between the composite and dentine. It is important not to over-dry the dentine after etching and the composite core should be built up in small layers to prevent contraction. If the tooth requires a crown then the glass ionomer or composite restoration can be used as a core.

If more tooth substance is lost then cutting an access cavity for root canal treatment severely weakens the tooth, and a crown may be necessary. The classic situation is that of an anterior tooth with mesial and distal restorations that have the radiographic appearance of an 'apple core' of remaining tooth substance. Cutting an access cavity removes the remaining spine of dentine, thereby weakening the remaining tooth substance.

EXTENSIVE RESTORATION

When an anterior tooth is severely broken down, discoloured or heavily restored with plastic materials, a full crown needs to be made.

CROWNS

Crowns with Metal Substructure

Metal–Ceramic Crowns

Metal–ceramic crowns are very strong and resist occlusal loads well. Minimal preparation (0.5 mm) is required on the palatal and approximal surfaces. This may be beneficial in a root-filled tooth with little remaining coronal tooth substance. The buccal surface, however, requires more tooth reduction (1.0–1.5 mm) than a porcelain jacket crown (0.8–1.0 mm). Inadequate tooth reduction can lead to a bulky crown and poor aesthetics. It is possible to finish the buccal margins with a porcelain butt shoulder to improve the marginal fit and give excellent appearance (Fig. 9.9).

Metal–Composite Crowns

Metal–composite crowns are often used as long-term provisional restorations. The composite discolours with time.

Metal-Free Crowns

Porcelain Jacket Crown

Porcelain jacket crowns require a buccal tooth reduction of between 0.8 and 1.3 mm, and can therefore be more conservative on tooth substance than a metal–ceramic crown. Stained dentine and metal posts affect the aesthetic appearance of a porcelain jacket crown; however, they can be placed over cores built up in

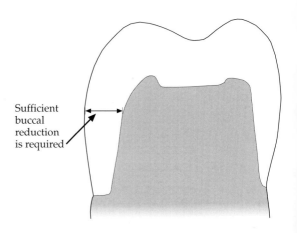

Sufficient buccal reduction is required

Figure 9.9

During crown preparation, sufficient buccal reduction of tooth substance is required.

composite or glass ionomer. Excessive occlusal loading may be a problem and can result in unpredictable fracture. In-ceram crowns have a glass infiltrated aluminium oxide ceramic core covered with conventional porcelain. Greater tooth reduction is required than with a metal–ceramic crown (1.5–2.0 mm for In-ceram crowns). By using a composite core, excellent aesthetics can be achieved. The Empress system uses heat and pressure to form a leucite glass–ceramic. A tooth reduction of 1.5–2.0 mm is required for Empress crowns. These crowns may be contraindicated in cases where there is evidence of excessive occlusal loading. The Procera technique uses computer-aided design and manufacturing technology to cut the core from an aluminium oxide block. The core is then coated in porcelain in the laboratory. Tooth reduction is similar to that of a metal–ceramic crown, but the laboratory costs are considerably greater.

ANTERIOR TEETH REQUIRING AUXILIARY RETENTION

If there is insufficient coronal tooth tissue remaining for retention of the crown then a post and core is required.

Posts

A post purely increases the retention of the core and crown; it does not strengthen the tooth. The choice of post is frequently empirical and the evidence base for selection is rather poor. A post that fits the remaining tooth substance should therefore be used, rather than adjusting the tooth to fit the post.

Shape

The shape of the post is dictated primarily from the space provided by the root canal. Preparation should be conservative, so as not to weaken the tooth unnecessarily by excessive removal of dentine. Posts can be parallel-sided, tapered or custom-made cast posts. Generally parallel-sided posts provide better retention than tapered posts, and although

they produce greater hydraulic forces during cementation, they perform better during function. Tapered posts can create wedging forces when occlusal loads are applied (Figs. 9.10 and 9.11).

Length

In order to maintain an adequate seal there must be at least 4 mm of root canal filling material present apical to the post. The size, length and curvature of the root also dictates the length of a post.

Many rules have been recommended as to the ideal length of the post. However, there is little clinical evidence to provide guidance. There is some indication, however, that a post

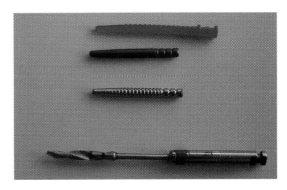

Figure 9.10

The Tenax (Whaledent, Mahwah, NJ, USA) titanium post kit (top to bottom): a wax burnout post, aluminium temporary post, titanium preformed post and a post drill.

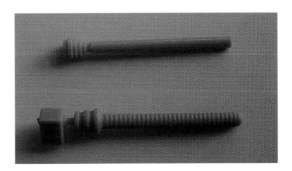

Figure 9.11

(Top to bottom) An impression post and a wax burnout post for a parallel, serrated post system.

should be at least as long as the crown that it supports and that in periodontally involved teeth the post should extend below the alveolar crest. The degree of occlusal loading affects the likely prognosis; a short post under a high stress would probably fail.

Diameter

The diameter of the post is again dictated by the root canal anatomy. Overpreparation in roots that are oval in cross-section or that have proximal external grooves results in perforation.

The post should be wide enough so that it does not deform under loading. This will depend on the alloy used for construction. A post should not be so wide that the root is unnecessarily weakened, since this increases the risk of root fracture (Fig. 9.12).

Surface Characteristics

Posts can be serrated, smooth, roughened or threaded. Parallel, serrated posts are cemented into the canal passively. They are retentive and produce less stress in the root dentine than threaded systems. A serrated parallel-sided post is usually the optimal choice for an anterior root-filled tooth. Smooth-sided cast posts are used in canals that are oval in cross-section or when there has been significant loss of coronal dentine from the root canal. The surface of the cast post can be sandblasted to improve retention. Ceramic posts are smooth and are used with a dentine bonding agent to improve retention. Cutting a venting channel along the length of serrated or cast posts with a carborundum disc or a fine long-tapered diamond reduces the hydraulic forces produced during cementing by allowing air and cement to escape coronally.

Threaded posts generate greater stresses within the root dentine. Pretapping the screw thread and avoiding overtightening reduces these forces (Fig. 9.13).

Parallel threaded posts can be useful in situations where there is limited root length available, perhaps as the result of an obstruction. Tapered threaded posts should be avoided since they produce wedging forces within the root canal that can result in fracture.

Material

Custom-made posts are often cast from gold or palladium alloys. Wrought posts are manufactured from stainless steel and titanium. Posts can also be made from carbon fibre and ceramic materials. Ceramic posts are more rigid than stainless steel posts, but tapering ceramic posts are less retentive than metal parallel serrated posts, even when used with a silane bonding agent.

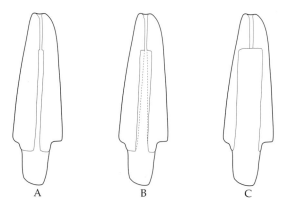

A   B   C

Figure 9.12

The diameter of the post is dictated by the remaining root substance and root canal space: (A) too narrow; (B) optimum size post; (C) too large.

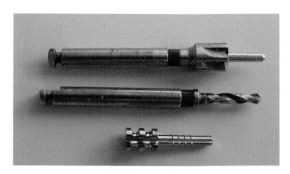

Figure 9.13

The Radix anchor post system (Maillefer, Ballaigues, Switzerland).

Post and Core Fabrication

If a post is required to restore an anterior tooth then a parallel serrated post that is preformed or cast is usually the first choice, taking into account the constraints of the remaining tooth substance and root canal space.

Preparation of the Post Hole

Post holes can be prepared immediately after root canal obturation, since this will not affect the quality of the seal. Gutta percha is removed to the desired depth using Gates-Glidden burs in a slow-speed handpiece. This creates a pilot channel for the post drill and helps to prevent perforation of the root canal wall. The post space can be prepared using a post drill and is rotated by hand or in a slow speed handpiece.

Using a Preformed Post

Serrated posts are cemented into the root canal using zinc phosphate cement, glass ionomer or a dentine bonding agent. Some posts are vented along the length of the post to reduce hydraulic forces and allow the escape of air and cement from the post hole. The core is then built up with light cured composite or glass ionomer. The composite is added in small increments to ensure complete polymerization and to prevent the adverse effects of contraction.

Indirect Cast Post and Cores

A small button is created on one end of the plastic post pattern. This is inserted into the root canal and an impression is taken. The post is removed with the impression. Cast post and cores are sometimes useful when multiple teeth are being restored. Casting porosity can lead to a risk of failure, which usually occurs at the junction between the post and core. A gradually tapering form between the post and core is recommended rather than a sharp junction between the two (Figs. 9.14 and 9.15).

Direct Cast Post and Core

An acrylic material such as Duralay (Reliante Dentaman, IL, USA) can be used to create a core in vivo, which can then be cast directly in the laboratory. The prepared dentine and post hole are brushed with a light coating of separating medium. A burnout post is inserted into the canal. The acrylic material is mixed and placed into position to build up the core. After the material has set, the core can be trimmed and occlusal reduction confirmed before casting is performed in the laboratory.

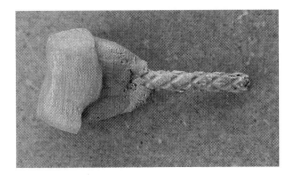

Figure 9.14

A cast core. There is a gradual junction between the post and core to distribute stresses more effectively.

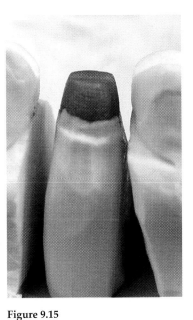

Figure 9.15

The post and core in situ on a stone die. The crown margins are on sound dentine.

Cementing the Post

The post space in the root canal is coated with cement using a spiral filler or endodontic file and the post is inserted. Pressure is applied until the cement is set. A venting groove prevents the post backing out of the canal as a result of hydraulic forces. It is preferable to apply cement to the canal rather than solely to the post, since in the latter case cement may be removed from the post on seating, resulting in poor bonding at the apical end of the post. Zinc phosphate, polycarboxylate and glass ionomers can all be used to cement metal posts. Chemically active resins such as 4-metaldehyde-based materials bond the metal to tooth substance and improve retention. Carbon fibre and ceramic posts are used with dentine bonding agents and chemically active resins.

POSTERIOR TEETH

Simple Restoration

If the remaining tooth is almost intact following endodontic treatment and there are no signs of cracking, then the access cavity can be filled using amalgam or light cured composite. An adequate coronal seal can be achieved by placing a zinc oxide and eugenol material (IRM) across the pulp floor and packing amalgam on top. When an adhesive system is used, a layer of IRM can be retained across the pulp floor; however, it must be covered with glass ionomer before light cured composite is placed, since the eugenol may inhibit the action of dentine bonding agents. An alternative solution is to use a thin layer of glass ionomer across the pulp floor and to bond directly to this. A light cured glass ionomer such as Vitrebond can be extremely useful for this purpose. If the tooth is to be restored with a glass ionomer or composite restoration, the access can be filled with glass ionomer immediately after completion of the root canal treatment, and a few millimetres can be cut back at a later appointment for the placement of a light cured composite. This allows maturation of the glass ionomer,

which does not need to be etched when placing the composite.

MESIO-OCCLUSAL CAVITIES

Plastic Restorative Techniques

The best method of restoring a root-treated tooth with an existing proximal box depends on the size and depth of the box and on the occlusal stresses that are applied during mastication. In a case with a shallow box and no evidence of occlusal loading, an amalgam restoration could be used. If, however, the tooth provides lateral excursive guidance or if there is evidence of cracking, then some form of cusp coverage cast restoration would be more appropriate.

It has been suggested that mesio-occlusal cavities could be restored with adhesive-style plastic restorations, but this has yet to be proven clinically. If there is a risk of cuspal flexing and tooth fracture, some form of cast cusp-coverage restoration is required.

CONSERVATIVE CUSPAL COVERAGE RESTORATIONS

If there are signs of cracks in the cusps of a tooth or across the marginal ridges then cuspal coverage and protection is required.

A bevelled margin of 1 mm depth is prepared around the circumference of the tooth. Base metal alloys can be bonded to the etched occlusal surface of the tooth using a silane bonding system. Extra retention will be provided by the internal contours of the access cavity, the majority of which is packed with IRM.

TEETH WITH MESIO-OCCLUSAL-DISTAL CAVITIES

When a tooth has two proximal boxes it is extremely important to protect the tooth from fracture.

Plastic Restoration

A capped cusp amalgam restoration can be used to protect the tooth from fracture. The cusps are reduced in height and the entire occlusal surface is rebuilt in amalgam. The technique is technically demanding since the correct occlusal contacts are difficult to achieve, and the material must be thick enough to withstand occlusal forces (2–3 mm). Direct light cured composite materials are not really suitable for use in this situation, and indirect composite or porcelain restorations have not yet been tested in long-term clinical follow up studies.

Cast Restorations

The most conservative cast restoration is the partial veneer onlay.

If a metal–ceramic crown is required, significantly more tooth substance will need to be removed (at least 1–1.5 mm). The clinician needs to be sure that sufficient tooth substance will remain after preparation for retention of the restoration to avoid an unnecessarily weakened tooth.

SEVERELY BROKEN-DOWN TEETH

Core Materials

Amalgam

Amalgam is often the material of choice as a core material on posterior teeth. It is strong and easy to use. Added retention can be gained by packing the amalgam into irregularities and undercuts in the pulp chamber and by using grooves, slots and pits in the cavity walls. Self-tapping dentine pins are rarely needed, and they may impart unwanted stresses within the dentine. Titanium rather than stainless steel pins may help reduce these stresses. The pins should be placed in sound dentine, well away from the future margins of any crown preparation. A bonding system may also provide increased retention as well as reducing coronal leakage.

Because amalgam has a slow setting reaction, crown preparation cannot always be carried out at the same visit (Fig. 9.16).

The Nayyar core

The Nayyar core is a useful means of restoring a molar tooth after root treatment when there is sufficient remaining tooth substance to support the core. Amalgam is packed into the root canals to a depth of approximately 3 mm and into the pulp chamber to give mechanical retention. An adhesive can be used to give extra retention (Fig. 9.17).

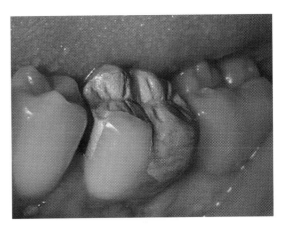

Figure 9.16

An amalgam core.

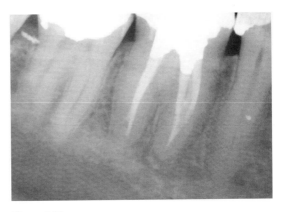

Figure 9.17

A Nayyar core. Amalgam has been packed into the coronal 2–3 mm of the root canals and the pulp chamber for added retention.

Composite

Composite cores have the advantage that they can be built up and prepared at the same visit. Chemically activated materials such as Ti Core (Essential Dental Systems, Hackensack, NJ, USA) have been shown to perform well. There is some concern in the literature that there may be risk of microleakage between the composite core and dentine (Figs. 9.18 and 9.19).

Cermets

Although cermets have been recommended as core materials they are not as durable as amalgam or composite. Cermets such as Ketac Silver (ESPE) are easy to use and bond to tooth substance. They should not be used when strength is required, but they could be used as a space filler to reduce the amount of alloy required in a cast restoration.

Cast cores

Complex cast cores with removable accessory posts are technically demanding to make and fit, and may be of little extra benefit compared with a well-placed amalgam core.

Using Posts in Posterior Teeth

Posts are rarely required in posterior teeth and do not add strength to the tooth. If a post is required then it should be placed in the largest canal. Posts are contraindicated in the minor canals of multirooted teeth. Preparation of the post space in these curved fine canals increases the risk of perforation, and the additional retention achieved is rarely advantageous over that provided by the pulp chamber and coronal aspect of the root canals. The post should ideally be parallel-sided and serrated. Venting grooves are cut in the post before cementation. Tapered screw posts (such as Dentatus: Tricare, Bradford, UK) are avoided as they place excessive stress on the walls of the root and may lead to fracture. The forces produced by parallel-sided screw posts (such as the Radix anchor) can be

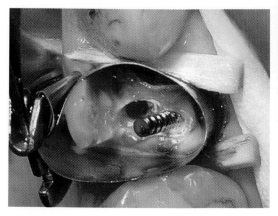

Figure 9.18

Building a composite core in a root-filled premolar. A titanium preformed post has been cemented into the buccal canal.

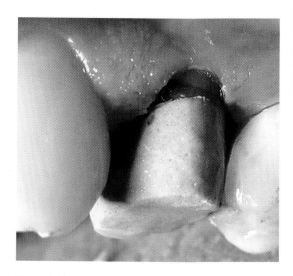

Figure 9.19

The completed core. Crown margins will be on sound dentine.

reduced by pretapping the screw thread and not tightening the post down hard.

Crowns for Posterior Teeth

The types of crown available for restoration of posterior teeth are similar to those discussed for anterior teeth, with the inclusion of cast metal crowns.

Cast Metal Crowns

High noble metal alloys are considered to be best since they have the greatest resistance to corrosion and tarnishing and are easy to work with.

Metal crowns are excellent in situations where the patient is not concerned with the appearance of metal. Significantly less reduction in the tooth is required to fit a cast metal restoration (0.5–1.0 mm) than for a metal–ceramic or ceramic restoration (1–2 mm).

Partial Cast Metal Crowns

Partial cast metal crowns may be used when the buccal surface of the tooth is intact. They are more conservative of tooth tissue than complete crowns, but they are more demanding technically both for clinician and in the laboratory (Figs. 9.20 and 9.21).

Full Cast Metal Crowns

The preparation for a full cast metal crown is more conservative than for a metal-ceramic crown (0.5–1.0 mm compared with 1.0–2.0 mm).

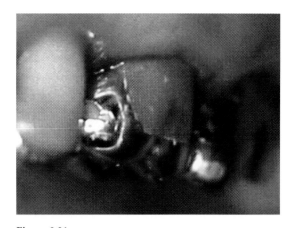

Figure 9.21

The cemented crown.

Metal–Ceramic Crowns

Metal–ceramic crowns are generally used when a patient requires a more aesthetic restoration. Porcelain can be used on the visible surfaces, such as the buccal and occlusal surfaces of mandibular teeth. If the clinical crown height is small, then retention grooves are cut in the core to provide added retention (Figs. 9.22–9.24).

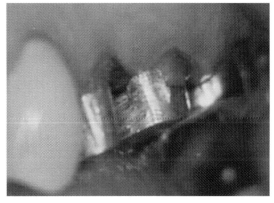

Figure 9.22

The maxillary second premolar and first molar have been prepared for metal–ceramic crowns. The teeth were restored with amalgam cores following root canal treatment. The crown margins are all on sound dentine, creating a ferrule effect.

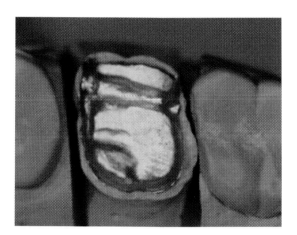

Figure 9.20

The stone die for a partial cast metal crown.

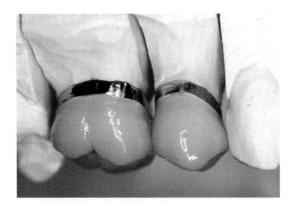

Figure 9.23

The crowns have metal margins for strength.

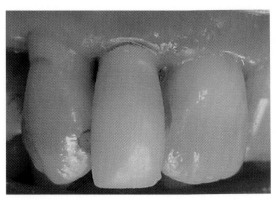

Figure 9.25

A custom cast acrylic temporary on a lateral incisor. The margins are well finished and the restoration is polished to improve the aesthetics and to prevent plaque accumulation.

- Custom-cast temporaries (Fig. 9.25).

For posterior teeth, temporary crowns include:

- Metal shell crown forms
- Custom-cast temporaries
- Long-term temporaries, metal–acrylic and metal–composite crowns.

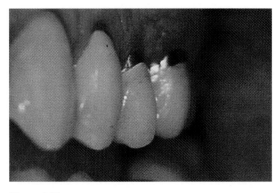

Figure 9.24

The cemented restorations.

Ceramic Crowns

Occasionally it is reasonable to use a castable or high-strength ceramic crown on a posterior tooth, if occlusal factors are not inhibitive. The amount of tooth reduction is more than with a metal–ceramic crown (occlusal reduction of 2 mm) and may compromise retention, especially in teeth with a short crown height.

TEMPORARY CROWNS

The types of temporary crown used depend on their location. For anterior teeth, temporary crowns include:

- Polycarbonate and acrylic temporary crown forms

Custom Cast Temporary Construction

Probably the simplest and most versatile method of producing temporary crowns is by casting custom-made restorations in an impression directly onto the prepared teeth.

The temporary crown material can be cast in an alginate impression taken before tooth preparation or a blowdown splint constructed from a plaster model. The latter method is very useful if the temporaries are to conform to a new occlusal relationship. The material is injected into the impression corresponding to the temporaries required. The alginate or blowdown splint is then fitted into the mouth and held in position until the material has started to set. Some clinicians advocate removing the material just before it becomes completely set and has a rubbery texture, since at this stage it is easier to remove from undercut areas. Any flash is trimmed from the margins and the crowns fitted with temporary cement. The surfaces and margins should be polished (Figs. 9.26–9.29).

ROOT-FILLED TEETH AS ABUTMENTS

Root-filled teeth and associated restorations tend to have a higher tendency to fail mechanically than vital abutments. Post-retained restorations fare less well as abutments for fixed bridgework or removable

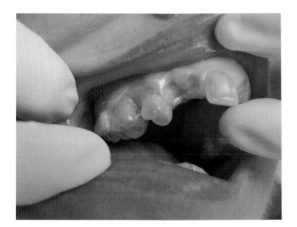

Figure 9.26

A vacuum stent can be used in complex cases if multiple temporaries are required.

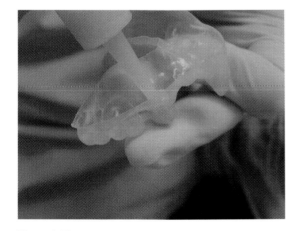

Figure 9.27

The temporary material is injected into the stent.

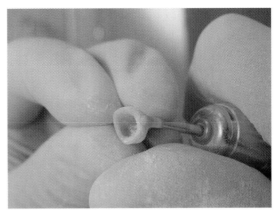

Figure 9.28

Flash is removed from the cast temporaries and the surfaces are polished.

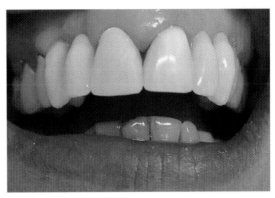

Figure 9.29

The cemented temporary restorations have excellent aesthetics.

prostheses than root-filled teeth without posts. This may be because the stresses distributed on root-filled abutment teeth are different from those applied to single unit restorations.

Ideally, root-filled teeth are avoided as abutments for bridges and removable prostheses. The forces applied to a fixed–fixed bridge are distributed equally; less force will be applied to the minor abutment by using a fixed–moveable design. The distal abutment for a free-end saddle prosthesis will have greater forces applied to it than the abutment adjacent to a bounded saddle.

RECEMENTING A CAST RESTORATION OR POST CROWN

When a cast restoration becomes decemented, the dentine of the tooth becomes covered in plaque. It is important to remove this before recementation, since it is full of bacteria and will adversely affect the quality of the bond. The crown preparation or post space should therefore be flushed with sodium hypochlorite before cementation to kill and dissolve any bacteria lining the walls.

FURTHER READING

Kanca J (1992). Resin bonding to wet substrate. I. Bonding to dentine. *Quintessence International* **22:** 39–41.

Kvist T, Rydin E, Reit C (1989). The relative frequency of periapical lesions in teeth with root canal-retained posts. *Journal of Endodontics* **12:** 578–580.

Saunders WP, Saunders EM (1994). Coronal leakage as a cause of failure in root canal therapy: a review. *Endodontics and Dental Traumatology* **10:** 105–108.

Saunders WP, Saunders EM (1996). Microleakage of bonding agents with wet and dry bonding techniques. *American Journal of Dentistry* **9:** 34–36.

Sorensen JA, Engleman MJ (1990). Ferrule design and fracture resistance of endodontically treated teeth. *Journal of Prosthetic Dentistry* **63:** 529–536.

Sorensen JA, Martinoff JT (1984). Intracoronal reinforcement and coronal coverage: a study of endodontically treated teeth. *Journal of Prosthetic Dentistry* **51:** 780–784.

Sorensen JA, Martinoff JT (1985). Endodontically treated teeth as abutments. *Journal of Prosthetic Dentistry* **53:** 631–636.

Torabinejad M, Ung B, Kettering JD (1990). In vitro bacterial penetration of coronally unsealed endodontically treated teeth. *Journal of Endodontics* **16:** 566–569.

10 COMPLEX ENDODONTIC PROBLEMS

CONTENTS • Introduction • Assessment of Success or Failure • Surgical Endodontics • Perio-Endo Lesions • Resorptions of Tooth Substance • Further Reading

INTRODUCTION

After conventional root canal treatment has been carried out the clinician must be able to assess whether it has been successful. The patient's symptoms should have resolved and any periapical lesion that was present should start to resolve. Sometimes, difficult endodontic problems require combined treatment, with perhaps a surgical endodontic approach, periodontal treatment or long-term review. This chapter discusses the indications and treatment of complex endodontic problems, including:

- Assessment of success or failure
- Surgical endodontics
- Perio-endo lesions
- Resorptions of tooth substance.

ASSESSMENT OF SUCCESS OR FAILURE

Success or failure in endodontic treatment is assessed using many criteria, including resolution of the patient's symptoms, reduction in swellings, healing of sinus tracts, and radiological evidence of bony healing.

Patient's Symptoms and Signs

Following root canal treatment the clinician normally expects resolution of the patient's symptoms and signs:

- The patient should be pain-free
- Tenderness on palpation and percussion and discomfort in the buccal sulcus should all be relieved
- There should be evidence of healing of any sinus tracts
- No swelling adjacent to the offending tooth should be visible.

Radiological Evidence of Bony Healing

Comparison of preoperative and postoperative radiographs taken at intervals after treatment is used to assess success or failure. Conventional criteria for assessment are:

- Success – the width and contour of the periodontal ligament is normal or slightly widened around extruded filling material
- Uncertain – the size of a periapical lesion has decreased but has not disappeared
- Failure – periapical radiolucency persists; the existing lesion has remained unchanged or has enlarged.

Scientific studies have shown that it is possible to predict the outcome of treatment as early as 1 year after treatment; however, the accuracy of this assessment becomes greater at 2 years, and up to 4 years may be required in some cases to reach a stable outcome.

Most healing occurs within the first year of

treatment; those teeth that demonstrate partial healing in the first year are likely to heal eventually. At 2 years most teeth should have healed. If a tooth has shown definite signs of healing at this stage then prolonged observation is not normally required. However, those teeth that do not show signs of healing at 2 years may need to be reviewed for a further 2 years. To compare radiographs effectively, a standardized technique must be used to ensure similar angulation, position and magnification between radiographs. The paralleling technique of using a film holder and a beam-aiming device is therefore always recommended in endodontics.

Radiological Review

When?

- Immediately after root canal treatment
- 1 year after treatment
- 2 years after treatment – stop if healed
- 3 years after treatment – only if not healed
- 4 years after treatment – only if not healed.

SURGICAL ENDODONTICS

In modern endodontics there are relatively few indications for endodontic surgery. Indeed many of the historical indications (such as broken instruments, tightly curved canals and the presence of a cyst) are now usually obsolete. Studies comparing the effectiveness of endodontic surgery with root canal treatment have clearly shown a much higher success rate with conventional root canal treatment. The main cause of failure in surgically treated cases is the inability or failure to address the basic aetiological problem: bacterial infection of the root canal system.

When?

Endodontic surgery is therefore considered when:

- Conventional root canal treatment or retreatment has been carried out but has not been successful
- There is a strong possibility of failure with further nonsurgical treatment
- Biopsy of a lesion is indicated
- The root surface requires direct exploration under good illumination and magnification (as in cases of suspected longitudinal root fracture) (Fig. 10.1).
- Dismantling of a complex restoration or bridge is contraindicated (uncommon).

There are very few contraindications to surgery. The psychological and systemic condition of the patient must be assessed, and the experience and expertise of the clinician will define whether the patient may need to be referred. Few cases therefore are not amenable to surgery, certainly by the specialist with experience in surgical endodontics. Systemic conditions that may preclude surgery include:

- Severe uncontrolled hypertension
- Infective endocarditis
- Severe asthma
- Uncontrolled diabetes

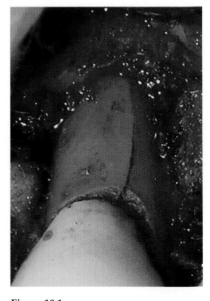

Figure 10.1

A longitudinal root fracture exposed by a surgical approach.

- Adrenal insufficiency or corticosteroid therapy
- Organ transplant
- Recent myocardial infarction
- Impaired hepatic or renal function
- Coagulation defects or therapy.

Surgical intervention may be required for incision and drainage, apical surgery and reparative or corrective surgery.

Incision and Drainage

Incision and drainage may be required when a patient presents with an acute apical abscess and fluctuant swelling in the buccal sulcus. Local anaesthesia is required.

Cortical trephination is a technique in which the cortical plate is punctured with a fine instrument (usually rotary) to try to achieve drainage. This is not an easy task to perform and there is a high chance of causing damage to the underlying root; it is not to be recommended.

Treatment of the acute abscess is covered in Chapter 12.

Apical Surgery

Apical Curettage

Periradicular curettage involves removing any pathological soft tissue from around the apex or lateral surfaces of the root end. The cementum at the apex of the root may be curetted and excess filling material removed. If tissue is required for biopsy, care must be taken to try and remove the lesion intact. The tissue to be examined is then placed in a suitable transport medium (such as 10% formol saline) and sent for histological evaluation. Any tissue removed during apical surgery should normally be assessed histologically.

Root-End Surgery

Curettage is rarely carried out without root-end surgery, since an attempt should be made to remove any residual infection that may be present inside the tooth. Root-end surgery requires the removal of the apical portion of the root, preparation of a root-end cavity and placement of a sealing root-end filling.

Corrective Surgery

Perforation Repair

Occasionally it is not possible to repair a perforation effectively using conventional root canal treatment techniques. The three factors that are important in the successful treatment of perforations are:

- The time since occurrence
- The size of the perforation
- The position relative to the crestal bone level.

Root Resection

Root resection consists of the removal of an entire root from a multirooted tooth without removal of the corresponding portion of the crown. It may be required when a particular root has had gross periodontal destruction around it, when there has been extensive inflammatory resorption or when there is a vertical root fracture.

Tooth Resection

In a tooth resection, the root and corresponding coronal tooth structure is removed. The separated part of the tooth may be retained and restored individually or removed.

The Surgical Armamentarium

A normal layout for a surgical procedure includes:

- Local anaesthetic syringe
- Aspiration tips
- Gauze swabs
- Cotton wool rolls and pellets
- Container for sterile saline
- Specimen pot and 10% formal saline

- Micro scalpel blades
- Periosteal elevator
- Periosteal retractors
- Probes
- Front surface mirror
- Micro mirror
- College tweezers
- Rat tooth tissue forceps
- Surgical handpiece (slow-speed or high-speed, or both)
- Burs for surgical handpiece
- Bone curettes
- Periodontal curettes
- Ultrasonic handpiece
- Specialist ultrasonic tips for root-end cavity preparation
- Carver, condensers and burnishers
- 4–0, 5–0 monofilament sutures
- Needle holders
- Surgical scissors
- Chlorhexidine mouthwash
- Root-end filling material (such as mineral trioxide aggregate (MTA: Dentsply, Weybridge, Surrey, UK), Super EBA (ethoxybenzoic acid: Staident International, Staines, UK) or Intermediate Restorative Material (IRM: Dentsply).

Anaesthesia, Pain Control and Haemostasis

Good anaesthesia is obviously essential during surgical endodontics carried out on a conscious patient. Profound and long-lasting anaesthesia can be achieved using 2% lignocaine (lidocaine) with 1:80 000 adrenaline (epinephrine). The vasoconstrictor in such an anaesthetic prolongs the duration of anaesthesia and helps to induce haemostasis to provide a blood-free operative site. If a solution of 1:50 000 adrenaline is available, better haemostasis is achieved.

Anaesthesia for Procedures on Maxillary Teeth

Procedures on maxillary teeth usually require a combination of buccal and palatal infiltration. Nerve blocks of the greater palatine, sphenopalatine and superior alveolar nerves may also be required.

Anaesthesia for Procedures on Mandibular Teeth

Inferior dental nerve blocks are supplemented with buccal and lingual infiltration for procedures on mandibular teeth. Long buccal infiltration and mental nerve blocks are also useful.

Pain Relief

The administration of a nonsteroidal anti-inflammatory drug at least 1 hour before the surgical procedure should help to reduce postoperative discomfort. Some of the benefit may however be a 'placebo effect'. A single dose of 500 mg paracetamol or 400 mg ibuprofen should be sufficient.

Preoperative Mouthrinse

The patient is instructed to rinse thoroughly with a 2% chlorhexidine gluconate solution before surgery. This can be started 24 hours before surgery, or at the time of surgery before the local anaesthetic is administered. The mouthrinse reduces the number of bacteria in the mouth.

Flap Design and Reflection

Full Flaps

Full flaps can be described as horizontal, triangular, rectangular or trapezoid (Figs. 10.2, 10.3). For endodontic purposes the triangular flap is most appropriate in the posterior segments and the rectangular flap in the anterior segments. (The trapezoid design may disrupt the vasculature of the attached gingiva that runs in a vertical direction.)

Relieving incisions run across the attached gingiva and into the alveolar mucosa. Interdental papillae are retained intact and the relieving incision is normally started on the distal aspect of the papilla.

Flap reflection is started in the attached gingiva in the relieving incision, elevating the periosteum from the alveolar bone. The papillae can then be eased away from the teeth with little trauma.

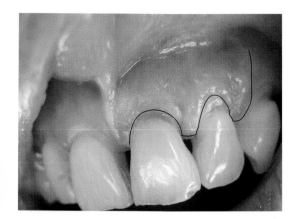

Figure 10.2

The outline of a triangular flap for surgery on the maxillary left lateral incisor.

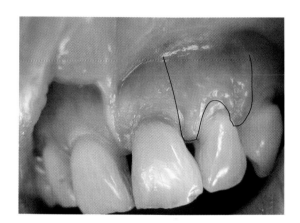

Figure 10.3

A rectangular flap for surgery on the maxillary left lateral incisor.

The flap is held away from the operative site with a retractor that is held firmly against the alveolar bone. The tissues must not become trapped between the elevator and bone since this can result in trauma to these delicate tissues.

Limited Flaps

Semilunar flaps in the alveolar mucosa give limited access and postoperative complications. They heal with scarring and are no longer recommended for endodontic surgery.

A Leubke-Ochsenbein flap in the attached gingiva does not impinge on crestal bone and can be useful in the anterior region when there is a wide band of attached gingiva and the teeth have been crowned. At least 2–4 mm of attached gingiva should remain between the gingival margin and the scalloped horizontal incision line. Scarring with this design of flap is not a serious problem (Figs. 10.4–10.6).

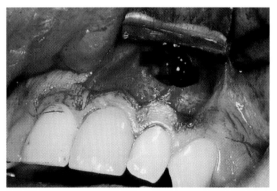

Figure 10.4

A Leubke-Ochsenbein flap.

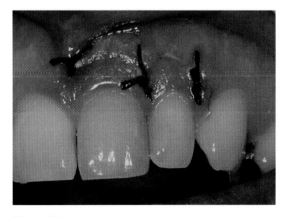

Figure 10.5

The Leubke-Ochsenbein flap 3 days following surgery.

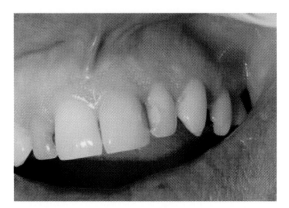

Figure 10.6

The surgical site after 2 weeks' healing.

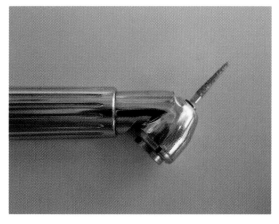

Figure 10.7

The Impact Air handpiece; the exhaust is directed away from the surgical site to prevent air embolism.

Osseous Entry

The bone around the apex of the tooth should be examined under good illumination and magnification. The cortical plate will be perforated if there has been a sinus tract. In many cases a sharp probe can be used to locate and identify the root apex and a curette used to peel away the cortical bone. The surgical site can then be modified if necessary with a slow-speed bur in a surgical handpiece with cold saline coolant or with a specialized high-speed surgical handpiece (Impact Air 45:

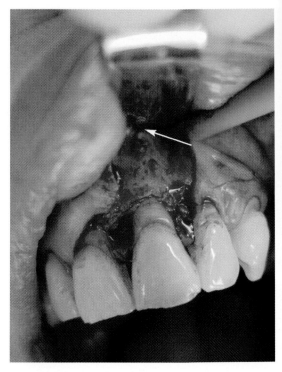

Figure 10.8

A chronic periapical lesion has perforated the cortical plate (arrow).

Palisades Dental, Piscatoway, NJ, USA) (Figs. 10.7 and 10.8). The lesion is excised using a curette and placed in 10% formol saline for histological evaluation.

Root-End Resection and Cavity Preparation

The apical 2–3 mm of the root is resected at a right angle to the long axis of the tooth (Fig. 10.9). (It is no longer considered appropriate to cut a bevel or to remove valuable root substance in order to gain access.) Microsurgical instruments are used to prepare the root-end cavity. These specialized tips are designed for use in a Piezon ultrasonic unit (EMS, Forestgate, Dallas, TX, USA) with irrigant. The tips are fine enough to prepare a cavity along the long axis of the root canal. Acoustic microstreaming produced during ultrasonic

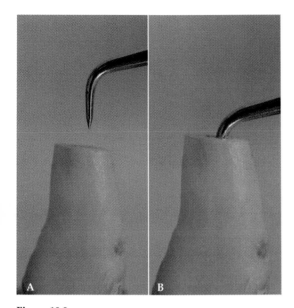

Figure 10.9

The root end is resected at right angles. Ultrasonic tips are used to prepare the canal along the axis of the tooth.

preparation helps to remove any bacteria that may be contaminating the root canal (Fig. 10.10).

Root-End Filling

- Good haemostasis must be achieved, and it may be necessary to place a cotton pledget containing vasoconstrictor in the bony cavity. The root-end cavity is dried using paper points and a fine air syringe (such as the Stropko syringe: Obtura Corporation, Fenton, MO, USA) and the root-end filling material is placed. The materials of choice are MTA, Super EBA or IRM. These are plugged into place (Figs. 10.11–10.13).

Postoperative Radiograph

It is important to take a postoperative radiograph before replacement of the tissue flap. This allows any necessary adjustments to be made.

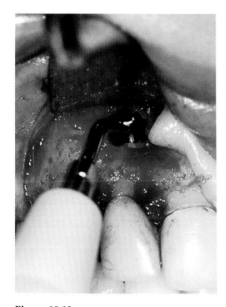

Figure 10.10

A Piezon ultrasonic tip being used to prepare a root-end cavity in a maxillary lateral incisor.

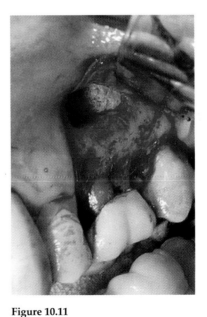

Figure 10.11

Cotton wool soaked in 1:1000 adrenaline has been packed into the bony cavity to achieve haemostasis.

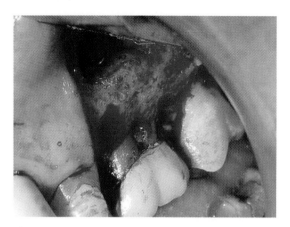

Figure 10.12

Mineral Trioxide Aggregate root-end fillings in the buccal roots of a maxillary first molar.

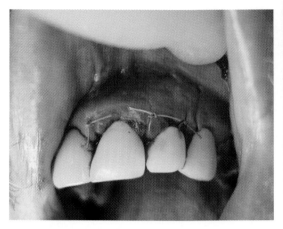

Figure 10.14

A triangular flap sutured with interrupted sutures.

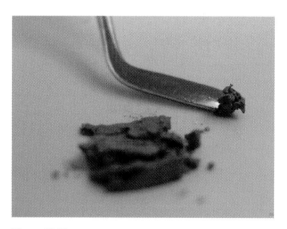

Figure 10.13

Mineral Trioxide Aggregate.

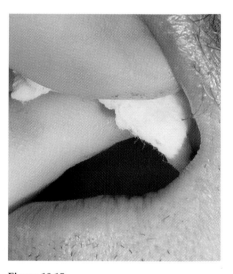

Figure 10.15

Pressure is applied to the flap following suturing.

Flap Replacement

The flap is returned to its original position and stabilized with sutures. Fine (4–0 or 5–0) monofilament sutures are probably best tolerated by the tissues. Firm pressure is then applied to the tissue flap with gauze soaked in saline for several minutes. This minimizes the size of the blood clot between the tissue and cortical bone, so that there will be less postoperative swelling and discomfort. The sutures are removed after 48–72 hours. Delay in suture removal often leads to gingival damage (Figs. 10.14 and 10.15).

Postoperative Instructions

The patient should be given the following instructions:

- Avoid strenuous activity, lifting heavy objects or sport for 24 hours
- Do not smoke
- Do not drink alcohol
- Eat soft foods and have hot drinks cooler than usual
- Do not be tempted to look at the surgeon's workmanship! This will pull unnecessarily on the tissue flap
- Slight bruising and swelling can be expected but should be minimal
- Take analgesics for up to 24–48 hours
- For the first few hours after surgery an ice pack should be applied to the face. This will reduce swelling
- A chlorhexidine mouthwash should be used three times a day starting 24 hours after surgery
- Teeth in the remaining quadrants can be brushed normally, but avoid the surgical site until the sutures have been removed
- Sutures should be removed after 48–72 hours.

Patients should also be given an emergency telephone number.

PERIO-ENDO LESIONS

In teeth with perio-endo lesions, either an endodontic lesion mimics periodontal disease or vice versa. In a few cases both endodontic and periodontal disease are present.

Although there are numerous connections between the periodontal ligament and the root canal (the apical foramen, lateral canals, furcal canals and a few dentinal tubules), there is little evidence that root canals become infected following the removal of cementum during periodontal debridement and root planing. Dentine has been shown to have a lower permeability to bacterial toxins than was previously thought. Periodontal disease is unlikely to affect the pulp even after the loss of tooth substance in the furcation following root planing.

Diagnosis

There are three main aids to the diagnosis of perio-endo lesions:

1 Good clinical examination, including periodontal probing
2 Pulp vitality testing
3 Good radiographs taken with a paralleling technique.

Periodontal Probing

Does the patient have evidence of marginal periodontitis around several teeth or is the periodontal condition generally good? This may give an initial indication as to the likely source of the problem around a particular tooth.

The periodontium around the tooth is gently probed using a fine tipped probe (0.5 mm and force of 25 g). Periodontal lesions tend to have a broad base whereas lesions of endodontic origin tend to result in a sudden increase in periodontal probing depth. A very deep but narrow pocket on opposite sides of a tooth may indicate a vertical root fracture.

The teeth can be grouped into one of three categories:

1 Teeth with a lesion of endodontic origin
2 Vital teeth with marginal periodontitis
3 Nonvital teeth with marginal periodontitis.

Pulp Vitality Testing

The pulp can be tested as described previously, using electric pulp testers or cold and hot stimuli. If a vital response is obtained from the pulp, the clinician may assume that the lesion is of periodontal origin, particularly with a single-rooted tooth. If the tooth is non-vital then the assumption is that there is an endodontic problem. If the tooth is not root filled or if the root filling is of poor quality, then root canal treatment or retreatment should be carried out. If the root filling is of very good quality, then periodontal treatment is required.

Paralleling Radiographs

The whole tooth must be visible on any diagnostic radiograph, the image must be clear and of adequate contrast, and there must be no elongation or foreshortening. The Rinn holder (Dentsply) allows the use of the paralleling technique, in which the film is held in a holder and the beam-aiming device ensures that the X-rays run perpendicular to the film.

The clinician must look for evidence of periapical radiolucency or of radiolucency adjacent to a lateral canal; this is most likely to be due to endodontic infection. Horizontal bone loss is found in periodontal disease. A pear-shaped radiolucency that follows the contour of the root is often associated with vertical root fractures.

Treatment

Correct treatment depends on accurate diagnosis, which involves thorough examination and testing. Treatment may be endodontic or periodontal, or both. If the prognosis is poor then the clinician must decide whether to proceed with the indicated treatment, whether to extract the tooth or perhaps whether to carry out root amputation or hemisection of the tooth. A 'try and see' approach to the treatment of perio-endo lesions is no longer appropriate. Successful treatment is based on a methodical approach to diagnosis (Fig. 10.16).

RESORPTIONS OF TOOTH SUBSTANCE

Several different types of pathological root resorption are recognized, and it can be difficult for the clinician to differentiate between them. Resorption can be classified into two types: internal and external. (External resorptions, except cervical resorption, are covered in Chapter 11.)

Internal Resorption

Internal resorption (Figs. 10.17–10.19) results from inflammation within the pulp. The pulp

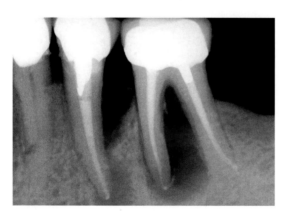

Figure 10.16

In this case the second premolar was nonvital and had both endodontic and periodontal lesions associated with it. The first molar was vital and therefore the origin of the lesion was periodontal; however, elective root canal treatment was carried out so that the mesial root could be resected.

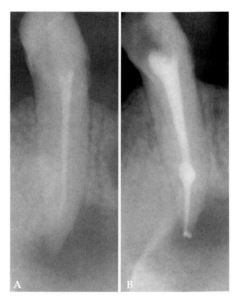

Figure 10.17

A case of internal resorption in a mandibular canine. (A) The patient presented with inadequate root canal treatment. (B) The canal system was retreated, irrigated throughly and filled with gutta percha.

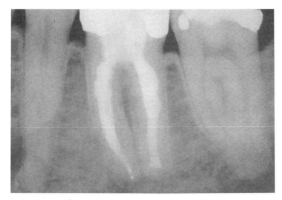

Figure 10.18

Internal resorption can occur in any tooth such as this molar.

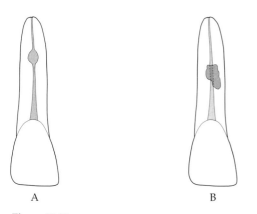

Figure 10.19

(A) Internal and (B) external resorption. In radiographs of external resorption the root canal is often still visible, superimposed over the resorption defect. In internal resorption the internal canal shape is altered.

is vital when the resorption is active, and the condition is often asymptomatic. Radiologically, the lesion has a smooth outline and appears as ballooning of the existing root canal. The pulp of the tooth may later become necrotic. Odontoclastic activity is triggered within the root canal, possibly following trauma or infection. This form of resorption is most common in incisor teeth but may occur in any tooth. The activity of the lesion is not continuous.

Diagnosis

The diagnosis of internal resorption is indicated by the following features:

- Vitality testing usually gives a positive response
- The lesion has a smooth border that merges with the outline of the root canal
- An angled radiograph shows the lesion centred on the pulp space
- Probing at the cervical margin does not reveal a defect.

Treatment

Conventional root canal treatment should be started immediately. The pulp of the tooth may haemorrhage during root canal treatment, and bleeding may be difficult to control. Ultrasonic irrigation is invaluable for cleaning the irregularly shaped root canal. A solution of sodium hypochlorite is used to dissolve the organic material within the root canal and to kill any micro-organisms. Haemorrhaging ceases when the pulp tissue has been completely removed. The root canal wall should be checked for perforation. This can be carried out using direct vision with good illumination and magnification, and also with an apex locator.

After canal cleaning and shaping, the canal is packed with calcium hydroxide as a temporary dressing between appointments. Owing to its high pH, this material is antibacterial and also helps to dissolve any remaining organic material.

The root canal treatment can usually be completed at a second visit. The irregular shape of the root canal is best obturated using a warm, vertically compacted gutta percha technique.

If the root canal is perforated referral may be indicated. On rare occasions large perforations may require surgical repair, but access is often extremely difficult.

Cervical Resorption

Cervical resorption (Figs. 10.20–10.22) may occur in the cervical region of a tooth following

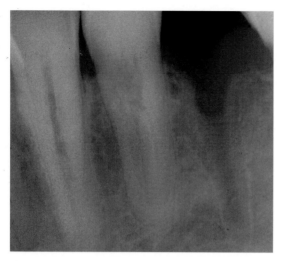

Figure 10.20

Burrowing external cervical resorption.

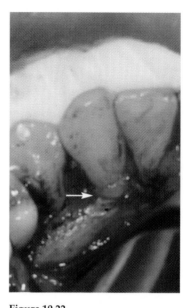

Figure 10.22

A cervical resorption defect exposed surgically on the lingual surface of a mandibular canine (arrow).

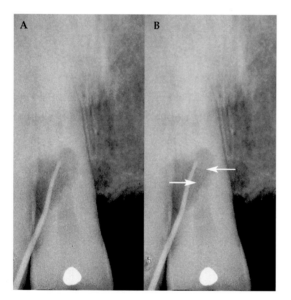

Figure 10.21

External cervical resorption. The root canal is still visible (arrows in B) superimposed over the defect.

trauma, including replantation of teeth. It is sometimes seen after a canine has been removed from the palate and transplanted, as a result of the trauma of extraction. It is localized external resorption caused by

inflammation within the periodontal ligament. Trauma such as aggressive scaling could possibly lead to odontoclastic activity in the cervical region of the tooth.

Clinically there may be a shallow crater subgingivally or the resorption may be of a burrowing form. The tooth is usually asymptomatic, and the pulp is vital and not part of the disease process. The resorptive process avoids exposing the pulp.

Diagnosis

The diagnosis of cervical resorption is indicated by the following features:

- The lesion is usually subgingival and detectable with a Briault probe; it must not be confused with a carious lesion
- The tooth is vital to electric pulp testing and thermal stimuli
- Radiologically there is an irregular radiolucency in the cervical region of the tooth; the root canal is intact
- If two radiographs are taken at different horizontal angles the defect appears to

move in relation to the root canal; this differentiates the lesion from an internal resorption
- In the later stages a pink spot may be observed in the coronal tooth substance.

Treatment

If the lesion is small and accessible, it should be surgically exposed, a cavity prepared and a restoration inserted. Light cured composite resin can be used. Lesions may sometimes recur. If the lesion is large or inaccessible then the tooth may need to be extracted.

FURTHER READING

Carr G, Bentkover SK (1998). Surgical Endodontics. In: Cohen S, Burns RC, eds. *Pathways of the Pulp*, 7th edition, Mosby, St Louis: 608–656.

Heithersay GS (1999). Clinical, radiologic, and histopathologic features of invasive cervical resorption. *Quintessence International* **30:** 27–37.

Ørstavik D (1996). Time-course and risk analyses of the development and healing of chronic apical periodontitis in man. *International Endodontic Journal* **29:** 150–155.

Simon JHS, Werksman LA (1994). Endodontic–periodontal relations. In: Cohen S, Burns RC, eds. *Pathways of the Pulp*, 6th edition, Mosby, St Louis: 513–530.

Torabinejad M, Chivian N (1999). Clinical applications of Mineral Trioxide Aggregate. *Journal of Endodontics* **25:** 197–205.

11 ENDODONTIC CARE OF PERMANENT TEETH IN CHILDREN

CONTENTS • Introduction • Isolation for Endodontic Treatment • Trauma • Root Resorption • Management of Carious Teeth • Endodontic Treatment of Molar Teeth in Children • Teeth of Abnormal Form • Further Reading

INTRODUCTION

This chapter will cover endodontic care of permanent teeth in children, trauma (which is more common in children) and management of tooth malformations.

The most significant characteristic of permanent teeth in children is their immaturity. Development is not complete until several years after eruption, and although teeth are generally fully formed approximately 6 years after eruption, the process of maturation continues throughout life, as secondary dentine is laid down by odontoblasts. Young teeth have large pulp chambers, wide root canals and thin-walled roots. They also have wide dentinal tubules. Once pulpal vitality is lost, all maturation ceases. This leaves an immature tooth with a short root, thin fragile walls and a large pulp space that is readily contaminated by bacteria, which can enter through exposed dentinal tubules. Immature, pulpless incisors are very prone to cervical fracture and are often unsuitable for restoration with posts.

The main aim of care should be to preserve the vitality of the pulp, thereby allowing maturation to continue. The vitality of the pulp may be threatened by bacteria following trauma, and by microleakage via a carious lesion or leaking restoration. In each case the aim of treatment should be the same − to prevent the entry of bacteria or their toxins into the pulp, which results in loss of vitality and cessation of maturation. In assessing a damaged tooth it is therefore essential to ascertain whether or not the pulp is vital or capable of recovery. It is rarely necessary to remove the pulp immediately. Unless there are obvious signs of infection, time can be taken to reassess, and if in doubt it is better not to remove the pulp.

ISOLATION FOR ENDODONTIC TREATMENT

Isolation for endodontic treatment has been covered in Chapter 4, but children may present particular problems with partially erupted teeth. Most children accept rubber dam application if it is carefully explained and if adequate local anaesthesia is used.

Suitable clamps for children include the Ash A or 14A (Dentsply, Weybridge, Surrey, UK) for partially erupted molars and the Hygenic 8 for slightly more erupted teeth. An Ash EW clamp fits most other teeth.

Sometimes it is not possible to clamp the tooth being treated, such as when it is partially erupted, crowded or badly fractured. In these cases it may be helpful to use two or more confluent holes to include adjacent teeth and to clamp one or both of these. This may leave a gap in the dam palatally, which can be sealed with Oraseal caulking (Ultradent, South Jordan, UT, USA) or a light-bodied impression material to prevent irrigant from entering the mouth. Local anaesthesia, including palatally if necessary, makes placement of a clamp much easier. In the mixed dentition stage the first premolar may be the most suitable tooth for clamping. A clamp can be placed over a fixed orthodontic appliance, or alternatively the arch wire should be removed by the orthodontist. Very occasionally it is really not possible to use a clamp; then it may be helpful to wedge a small portion of rubber dam or a Wedget (Hygienic, Akron, OH, USA) between two teeth, or alternatively to tie dental tape around the neck of the tooth.

An alternative method of isolation for anterior teeth is the Dry Dam (SDI Svenska Dental Instruments, Uplands Vasby, Sweden) (Fig. 11.1), which fits around the patient's ears and is used without a clamp. This can be a great advantage in very anxious patients, especially since it does not require the use of local anaesthesia. It is also very quick and easy to apply.

TRAUMA

Traumatic injury can result in fractures of the crowns and roots of teeth, luxation and avulsion injuries. Treatment should aim to preserve pulp vitality whenever possible.

General Considerations

• Was the patient unconscious? If so seek medical advice

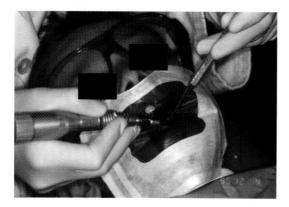

Figure 11.1

The use of dry dam for isolation.

• Are there other injuries? Bone and soft tissue damage should be assessed. Lacerations and fractures require immediate attention and take precedence over dental trauma. It may be necessary to seek specialist advice
• Is there any relevant medical history?
• What is the patient's tetanus status?

Things to look for include:

• What is the nature of the injury?
• Are the damaged teeth restorable?
• Has there been a previous dental injury? This may confuse the diagnosis
• What is the likely prognosis?
• What will the overall treatment plan involve?
• Has the vascular supply to the tooth been impaired or severed? This is particularly relevant in luxation injuries
• Is it likely that the pulp has been contaminated by micro-organisms? Micro-organisms can take many days to penetrate a significant distance into the healthy pulp in an immature tooth
• Is the root fully developed?

Note that immature teeth with large pulp spaces and thin root canal walls can be difficult to restore and are prone to fracture. Root-end closure procedures often take in excess of 1 year to complete.

Diagnosis

An accurate diagnosis is essential if mistakes and incorrect treatment are to be avoided. It can be particularly confusing when several teeth have received different injuries or when there has been a previous dental injury. It is therefore essential to take a careful and detailed history. Often a traumatized tooth does not respond to sensitivity testing during the first few months after injury, but this may be transient and therefore the pulp should not be removed on this evidence alone. There must be additional evidence that the pulp is infected before its removal is considered. If the prognosis of a traumatized tooth is poor, consideration should be given at an early stage to its eventual replacement. If the tooth is not restorable it may be extracted or the root may be retained to preserve alveolar bone.

Crown Fractures

Enamel or Dentine Fractures

Bacteria can enter the pulp through exposed dentinal tubules (resulting from a fracture into dentine) either immediately after the injury or at a later date. It is therefore essential when this injury occurs that the exposed dentine should be covered as promptly as possible to preserve the pulp. It is not always necessary to place a lining material over the exposed dentine, although many operators prefer to do this if the fracture is deep. An effective dentine bonding agent should be used, since the most important aspect of this treatment is the exclusion of infection. It is best to restore the tooth using etch-retained composite resin at the first visit. The tooth may be built up at a subsequent visit to restore both its anatomical relationship with the adjacent teeth and its appearance. Teeth should be monitored in case of later loss of vitality. A concomitant luxation worsens the prognosis.

Crown Fractures that Expose the Pulp

Things to look for include:

- A fracture that involves enamel and dentine
- Exposed pulp, with a red appearance, which indicates that the tooth is vital. If the pulp has a blue appearance in a tooth with a recent injury, this indicates that it is non-vital and is unsuitable for a pulpotomy
- Concomitant luxation injury.

Treatment

Partial Pulpotomy
Partial pulpotomy, as described by Cvek, is the treatment of choice. It has a very high success rate in immature teeth and a good record with mature teeth. The aims of partial pulpotomy are to:

- Remove damaged pulp tissue
- Seal the cavity to prevent microleakage.

The exposed pulp must be protected from contamination in order to preserve its vitality and allow continued maturation of the tooth. It has been shown that the size of exposure does not affect the outcome. Using local anaesthesia and rubber dam, a small cavity is cut at the exposure site, using a turbine bur with copious waterspray for cooling. This method is less traumatic than using a slow handpiece or excavators. It is important to cut the cavity to the level of vital healthy pulp tissue. The cavity should be washed using sterile saline, and haemorrhage should be controlled using sterile cotton pellets or large paper points.

A calcium hydroxide dressing is normally placed over the pulp. This dressing may be a setting variety such as Dycal (Dentsply) or calcium hydroxide powder mixed with water or sterile saline. Coronal seal is important. A fortified zinc oxide eugenol cement, such as IRM (Intermediate Restorative Material: Dentsply), still within the cavity, will give a good seal and also have an antibacterial effect (Fig. 11.2).

A layer of glass ionomer cement, such as Fuji IX (GC Corporation, Tokyo, Japan) prevents any interference with the setting of the

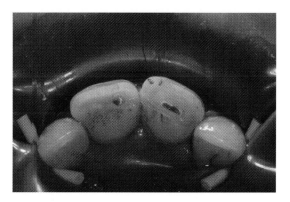

Figure 11.2

Partial pulpotomy; a cavity has been cut at the exposure site.

composite resin, which gives a final coronal seal. The cement should prevent contamination of the pulp if the composite restoration is lost (Fig. 11.3). Alternatively, mineral trioxide aggregate (MTA: Dentsply) may be used in the cavity and the tooth built up with composite resin. This pulp treatment induces formation of a dentine bridge, allowing the pulp to retain its vitality, the tooth to continue to mature and the root to grow (Figs. 11.4 and 11.5).

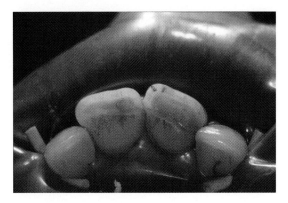

Figure 11.3

Glass ionomer placed over the dressing material to seal the pulpotomy cavity before placement of light-cured composite.

If the patient is very anxious or upset at the time of injury, it may be better to postpone the treatment for a day rather than compromise its quality. The tooth should be monitored clinically and radiologically at regular intervals (every 3–6 months).

If a fragment of tooth is to be reattached, this is done after the pulp treatment.

It cannot be stressed too strongly that if the pulp is vital it should NOT be removed. Successful pulpotomy should not be followed by root canal treatment.

Horizontal Root Fractures

Things to look for include:

- A tooth with abnormal mobility following trauma
- An upper standard occlusal radiograph showing evidence of a fracture line
- A radiolucency in the adjacent bone at the fracture line if the coronal fragment has become nonvital and infected.

Vitality testing may be unreliable for several months.

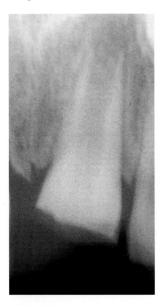

Figure 11.4

A radiograph showing a maxillary central incisor that has been treated by pulpotomy.

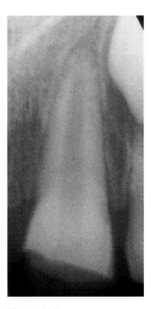

Figure 11.5

The same tooth as in Fig. 11.4 showing continued root development 16 months later.

Treatment

If the coronal portion is vital, treatment entails:

- Repositioning the coronal fragment (and splinting if indicated), soon after injury
- Observation.

If the coronal portion is nonvital and infected, treatment entails:

- Treatment of the coronal fragment as a nonvital tooth with an open apex
- Root canal treatment to the fracture line.

When a tooth sustains a horizontal root fracture the pulp normally remains vital; therefore its removal is contraindicated. If the fracture is near the apex and there is normal mobility, no active treatment is required. If there is abnormal mobility the coronal fragment should be splinted with a semirigid splint, usually for 2–3 weeks, but for up to 6 weeks if there is still excessive mobility.

If infection intervenes, the coronal fragment may become nonvital. The apical fragment remains vital almost without exception, and therefore any root canal treatment should be confined to the coronal portion. The coronal fragment may be so displaced that its blood supply is severed at the fracture line. In this case there is easy access for revascularization at the fracture line, and the coronal portion may regain vitality. It is therefore important not to remove the coronal pulp on the evidence of sensitivity testing alone. During healing there may be some remodelling resorption at the fracture line. This is part of the healing process and is not an indication for root canal treatment.

If there is also a coronal fracture, this predisposes to the ingress of bacteria and so the prognosis for pulp vitality may be worsened. Similarly, if the fracture line is close to the gingival sulcus, this can provide an entry for bacteria and so worsen the prognosis of the tooth. If a periodontal pocket communicates with a deeper fracture line, the prognosis for the coronal fragment of the tooth is very poor (Fig. 11.6).

A nonvital coronal fragment is treated in a similar way to a nonvital tooth with an open apex. Access is gained to the root canal of the

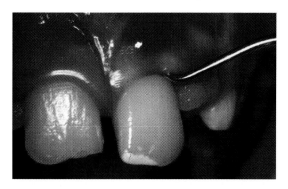

Figure 11.6

A deep periodontal pocket has developed following trauma; this indicates a poor prognosis.

coronal fragment using a sufficiently large access cavity to allow thorough cleaning. A radiograph is taken to assess the length to the fracture line. The canal is gently cleaned with files and irrigated with sodium hypochlorite. Calcium hydroxide is packed to the fracture line and replaced only when its density is seen on a radiograph to be reduced. When a hard tissue barrier has formed at the fracture line, the canal of the coronal fragment may be filled with gutta percha. Alternatively, when the infection is controlled and soft tissue healing has taken place, it may be possible to insert a 'plug' of calcium hydroxide at the fracture line and fill the remaining space with gutta percha (Fig. 11.7).

(A)   (B)   (C)

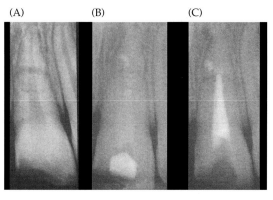

Figure 11.7

(A) A radiograph of a nonvital maxillary central incisor with a horizontal root fracture. (B) Calcium hydroxide has been inserted to the fracture line. (C) The tooth has been root filled to the fracture line.

If the coronal fragment is lost, a decision must be made as to whether or not sufficient root remains to restore the tooth. In a favourable situation the apical fragment could be extruded, or gingival surgery could performed to allow construction of a post crown. If this is not practical, it is often preferable to leave the fragment in situ to preserve the alveolar bone, unless there is infection or the space is required as part of orthodontic treatment.

Luxation Injuries

Following luxation injuries there is a possible route of infection via the damaged periodontal structures; therefore, after the tooth has been repositioned and, if indicated, stabilized, a strict regimen of chlorhexidine mouthwashes should be instituted. A concomitant crown fracture worsens the prognosis of the pulp because of possible ingress of infection via the dentinal tubules.

Concussion

Concussion is a periodontal ligament injury. The tooth becomes tender to pressure and there may be a temporary loss of response to sensitivity testing. The pulp is likely to remain vital.

Subluxation

In subluxation, the nerves and blood vessels that supply the pulp may be stretched or severed. Loss of vitality is unlikely but it can occur in mature teeth. Root resorption is rarely a complication.

Lateral Luxation

Lateral luxation is a more severe injury to the pulp, causing stretching, crushing or severance of the apical nerves and vessels. If the apex is open, revascularization is likely, followed by obliteration of the pulp space with hard tissue (Fig. 11.8). This dystrophic calcification is not an indication for root canal treatment, although the tooth may not respond to

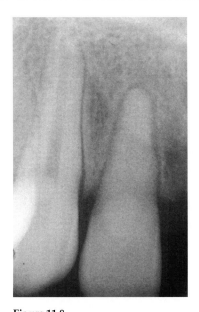

Figure 11.8

A tooth that was previously luxated and now shows calcification of the root canal.

sensitivity testing. If the apex is closed, pulp necrosis is more likely. However, it is worth waiting because of the possibility of healing after transient apical breakdown (see p. 185). Inflammatory or replacement resorption may occur later as a result of periodontal damage.

Extrusive Luxation

If extrusive luxation is severe, the blood vessels and nerve fibres may be severed. When the apex is open and there is no infection, there may be revascularization followed by pulp canal obliteration. If the apex is closed, necrosis is more likely. Inflammatory external root resorption is occasionally seen as a late complication.

Intrusive Luxation

Intrusive luxation causes a severe crushing injury to the periodontal ligament. Immature teeth may re-erupt spontaneously. In immature teeth there is a 30% chance of revascularization, whereas in mature teeth loss of vitality is almost certain and therefore root canal treatment is indicated. External inflammatory or replacement resorption is frequently a complication.

Transient Apical Breakdown

Transient apical breakdown has been considered to be nature's way of producing an open apex to allow regeneration of the pulp in mature luxated teeth. The tooth loses its blood supply and it may darken, cease to respond to sensitivity testing and even have an apical radiolucent area. If there is no intervention, some apical resorption may take place, followed by a return to normal colour, positive sensitivity testing and healing of any apical area. Frequently the pulp undergoes dystrophic calcification. Transient apical breakdown occurs in about 4% of mature luxated teeth.

Avulsion

When a tooth is avulsed, the blood vessels and nerve fibres entering the pulp are severed, as are the supporting periodontal fibres.

Emergency treatment involves cleaning the tooth if necessary, and then replacing it in its socket as soon as possible. This is best done at the site of the accident to reduce extraalveolar time. The tooth may be rinsed under cold running tap water.

If immediate replantation is not possible the tooth should be kept in a suitable transport medium; cold milk has been shown to be the best that is readily available. The patient should seek expert advice as soon as possible. It is the length of dry storage time that is most important for determining the prognosis of the tooth – the length of time in a suitable storage medium is less critical.

At the dental surgery it should be decided whether replantation is indicated; in this regard, consider the following points:

- Does the patient have a relevant medical condition? If the patient suffers from a bleeding disorder, an autoimmune disease or a congenital cardiac abnormality, is

immunosuppressed or has any other serious systemic disorder, consideration should be given as to whether replantation is appropriate, and if it is whether any special precautions should be taken. The clinician should consult contemporary guidelines and, if possible, the patient's physician
- The condition of the tooth – if the tooth has a very short root or is severely damaged, replantation may be contraindicated
- The age of the patient – in patients who are still growing, replantation may not be indicated because an ankylosed tooth would interfere with alveolar growth. The tooth would not erupt and would be in infraocclusion
- The extra-alveolar period and the storage medium – if the tooth has been dry for more than 1 hour, the cells of the periodontal ligament–cementum complex will have died and the tooth will later become ankylosed.

If replantation is to be performed at the surgery, the following points should be borne in mind:

- Local anaesthesia is always required for replantation, especially immediately after the accident
- Ask the patient to rinse first with a chlorhexidine mouthwash
- Clean the tooth gently using saline, preferably from a syringe, without handling the root
- Examine the socket and flush away the clot gently with saline
- Insert the tooth and press gently into the socket. If it will not seat correctly, re-examine the socket and, if necessary, gently reposition any fractured alveolar bone that is in the way
- The tooth should be splinted with a semi-rigid splint
- A radiograph should be taken to check the position of the tooth
- Tetanus prophylaxis is given if appropriate
- Chlorhexidine mouthwashes should be instituted from the next day.

After 7–10 days the splint is removed. If the tooth is mature it is assumed that the pulp will become necrotic and so it should be removed at this stage. The pulp space is disinfected and calcium hydroxide is inserted before definitive root filling.

If the tooth is immature it should be given time for possible revascularization. If revascularization occurs, the tooth will usually respond to sensitivity testing within 6 months, although some teeth take up to 2 years. External inflammatory resorption can occur very rapidly after replantation, and the tooth should be assessed radiologically during the first few months. If this or any other sign of infection is seen, the pulp should be removed and the pulp space promptly disinfected. This arrests inflammatory resorption. The tooth is treated as any nonvital immature tooth (Fig. 11.9).

The Nonvital Immature Tooth

A tooth that has lost its vitality at a young age is likely to have a doubtful prognosis, and this should be explained to the patient and the patient's parents at the outset. It may be useful to maintain such a tooth for a number of years while the child is growing and until an appropriate alternative can be provided.

The restorability of the tooth should be assessed at this stage to avoid prolonged treatment on a tooth that is not ultimately restorable. If the tooth is not restorable or has a poor prognosis it is not always necessary to extract it immediately. It may be more practical to wait until there is a problem before removing it and providing a replacement. If the tooth has a very poor prognosis, an early consultation should be arranged to plan for a replacement, which may be a bridge, a denture, an implant or a transplanted immature tooth.

Things to look for include:

- A history of trauma
- Signs of infection, such as pain, swelling or a sinus tract
- A tooth that is immature compared with antimere.

Treatment

Following isolation, an access cavity is cut incisal to the cingulum (larger than that in a mature tooth) in order to clean the wide root canal space effectively. If the tip of the tooth is restored, the access cavity may be extended to the incisal edge (Fig. 11.10) to improve access to the root canal. A balance must be sought between gaining adequate access and not weakening the neck of the tooth unduly, since it has been shown that these teeth are prone to cervical fracture. Because both sodium hypochlorite and calcium hydroxide dissolve organic matter it is not strictly necessary to have straight-line access to all parts of the canal. The most important aspect of treatment is to disinfect the root canal thoroughly with sodium hypochlorite. The working length is determined radiologically and the canal gently cleaned with files. The aim is to remove infected soft tissue, and not to file the already thin walls of the root. The canal is then dried and calcium hydroxide is inserted. Calcium hydroxide powder may be mixed with sterile water or saline; and one part in five barium sulphate may be added to increase radio-opacity. It is important to have a well-packed mass of calcium hydroxide in the root canal at the desired working length. The calcium hydroxide should be mixed to a thick putty consistency, which can then be packed into the root canal space using root canal pluggers. A plugger should be premeasured to the desired length and marked to a

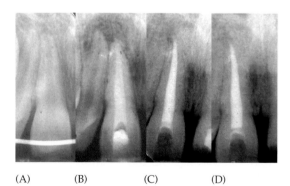

(A)   (B)   (C)   (D)

Figure 11.9

An avulsed maxillary incisor following its replantation and splinting (A). The tooth filled with calcium hydroxide (B). The same tooth showing the completed root filling (C). A successful outcome, 4 years after root treatment (D).

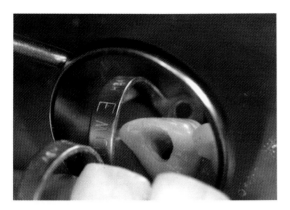

Figure 11.10

An access cavity for root canal treatment of an immature tooth. The cavity in the composite restoration has been extended to the incisal edge.

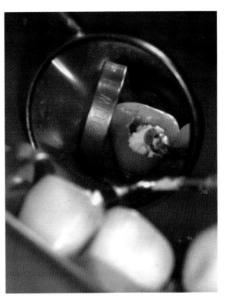

Figure 11.11

Placing calcium hydroxide in the access cavity with an amalgam plugger before finally packing the material with a root canal plugger.

reference point with a rubber stop. A small amount of calcium hydroxide putty should be put into the root canal and packed down to length (Fig. 11.11). If it is difficult to keep the canal dry because of apical inflammation, the putty will become slurry-like; a paper point should be used to draw water gently from the medicament. This makes it easier to pack the following section of putty.

Keep placing calcium hydroxide into the canal and gently pack into place until the canal is filled to the level of the cervical constriction. Alternatively, a proprietary nonsetting calcium hydroxide paste may be used, either by an injection technique such as Hypocal (Ellman International, New York, USA) thickened with calcium hydroxide powder or by insertion with a spiral filler. A temporary restoration of reinforced zinc oxide and eugenol, at the appropriate powder–liquid ratio is used to prevent coronal leakage.

When it is not possible to pack the calcium hydroxide thoroughly at the first visit, it should be replaced 1 or 2 weeks later. Normally it should be reviewed radiologically after 1 month and replaced if the density in the apical third is seen to have reduced. Thereafter it should be reviewed after approximately 3 months and then every 6 months; the calcium hydroxide should be replaced when necessary (and the canal irrigated with sodium hypochlorite).

In the early stages when the apex is wide open and there is apical inflammation, the calcium hydroxide may be seen to 'wash away' between visits. When the infection is brought under control, and a barrier is forming, it appears stable. A hard tissue barrier normally forms at the apex. The time taken for this to occur depends on the degree of immaturity of the tooth and the degree of infection at the beginning of treatment. It should form within 12 months (Fig. 11.12). There is no evidence of any advantage in delaying the permanent root filling until after completion of orthodontic treatment.

Troubleshooting Apical Barrier Induction

Failure to achieve a barrier may occur if:

- There is long-standing infection outside the tooth; surgery may be required in this case
- There is a vertical root fracture; although such a fracture is not always visible radiologically, there may be classical signs such

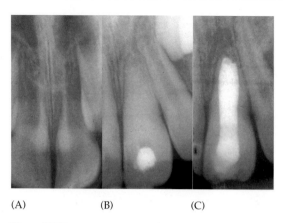

(A)   (B)   (C)

Figure 11.12

Nonvital maxillary central incisors in a young boy, aged 9 years (A). Calcium hydroxide has been packed into the canal and remains well condensed as apical growth continues (B). Completed treatment. The pulp space has been obturated with a gutta percha root filling (C).

hard tissue barrier has formed. As soon as there is soft tissue healing at the apex, the MTA is inserted into the apical few millimetres and gently condensed. A check radiograph is taken; if the filling is unsatisfactory it can be washed out immediately with water and then a new increment repacked. The material takes several hours to set. A cotton pellet is inserted into the rest of the canal and the access cavity is sealed. At a subsequent visit the rest of the canal may be back-filled with gutta percha.

If the neck of the tooth is thin and at risk of fracture and if the tooth is not suitable for a post, composite resin may be bonded into the cervical area to strengthen it. Using an acid etch technique and a dentine bonding agent, the light cured composite is added in small increments to ensure complete setting and effective bonding.

as periodontal inflammation. Teeth that have fractured vertically need to be extracted

- The root canal space has not been disinfected effectively
- Failure of temporary restoration has resulted in coronal leakage.

Filling the Root Canal

When a hard tissue barrier has formed at the apex a permanent root filling may be inserted. Many of these teeth have very wide, irregularly shaped canals that are not readily filled by lateral condensation. A variety of methods may be employed. Gutta percha points may be used upside down or rolled together as a custom-made filling. The most satisfactory method is to inject thermoplasticized gutta percha, such as with the Obtura system (Texceed Corporation, Costa Mesa, CA, USA). The canal is first lightly coated with sealer. The apical few millimetres are filled and the gutta percha is compacted using Machtou pluggers (Maillefer, Ballaigues, Switzerland). A check radiograph is taken and the rest of the canal is filled in increments.

Alternatively MTA may be used as a filling material, and it can be inserted before a

ROOT RESORPTION

Several different types of pathological root resorption are recognized and it can be difficult for the clinician to differentiate between them. Resorption can be classified as either internal or external. Internal resorption is covered in Chapter 10.

External Resorption

There are six groups of external resorption that affect the teeth of children:

- Surface resorption
- Inflammatory resorption
- Replacement resorption
- Pressure resorption
- Systemic-related resorption
- Idiopathic resorption.

Surface Resorption

Surface resorption usually occurs as the response to mild localized injury of the periodontal ligament and cementum. It is self-limiting and does not require treatment.

External Inflammatory Resorption

External inflammatory resorption (Figs. 11.13 and 11.14) is associated with the presence of damaged cementum and an infected pulp space. Toxins produced by the micro-organisms in the root canal system leave the root canal through dentinal tubules; they are covered by damaged cementum and stimulate osteoclastic activity. External inflammatory resorption of an immature tooth may progress very rapidly; therefore careful radiological observation is necessary in the early weeks after injury. Resorption is sustained by pulp infection. External inflammatory resorption occurs as a complication of severe luxation injuries.

Diagnosis

A diagnosis of inflammatory resorption is indicated by the following features:

- The tooth is nonvital to pulp testing
- There are radiological signs of destruction of the root of the tooth and adjacent bone, laterally or apically.

Treatment

Treatment must be instituted promptly, since destruction can be very rapid, and a large part of the root may be destroyed within weeks. This process is readily arrested by disinfection of the pulp space.

The pulp space should be cleaned and disinfected with sodium hypochlorite before placement of a calcium hydroxide dressing. When the infection has been controlled, healing will take place. A new periodontal ligament forms to surround the defect. A root filling may then be inserted when appropriate.

A variation of inflammatory resorption, cervical resorption, may occur in children after trauma. It is discussed in Chapter 10.

Replacement Resorption

Replacement resorption (or ankylosis) is the slow replacement of the root by bone. It results from damage to the cells of the cementum–periodontal ligament complex and classically occurs in teeth that have been replanted or transplanted or have suffered luxation injuries (Fig. 11.15).

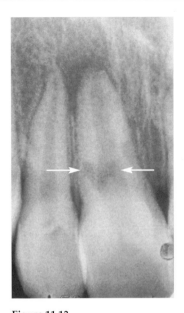

Figure 11.13

Early inflammatory resorption of maxillary central incisor (arrows).

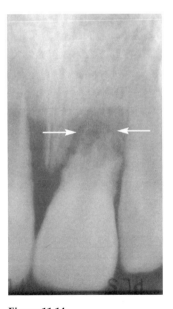

Figure 11.14

Advanced inflammatory resorption of a maxillary central incisor (arrows).

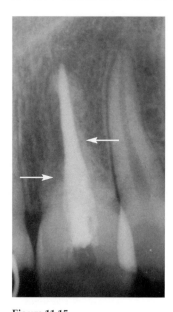

Figure 11.15

Replacement resorption of a maxillary central incisor (arrows).

Diagnosis

A diagnosis of replacement resorption is indicated by:

- A history of trauma
- A lack of physiological mobility
- A resounding ringing note when the tooth is tapped
- The tooth being in infraocclusion (which occurs sometimes)
- Radiologically a root that looks moth-eaten or irregular in outline with a loss of periodontal ligament space
- Absence of radiolucency in the surrounding bone.

The pulp may be vital or nonvital.

Treatment

Replacement resorption is not treatable; however, it may be minimized by careful management). If the tooth has both replacement resorption and inflammatory resorption associated with it, then disinfection of the root canal and dressing with calcium hydroxide may slow the rate of the inflammatory resorption. The patient should be warned that the tooth will ultimately be lost. This will occur more rapidly in young patients, in whom bone turnover is rapid. The tooth may be in infraocclusion and may need to be extracted for aesthetic reasons. In this case most of the root should be retained to preserve alveolar bone. In older patients, the tooth may be retained for many years. If the pulp is vital, pulp extirpation is not indicated.

Pressure Resorption

Pressure resorption is self-limiting and will repair after removal of the cause. It is sometimes seen when chronic or acute pressure has been applied to the tooth, as in orthodontic treatment or by an erupting tooth, an impacted tooth, a tumour or a cyst.

Systemic-Related Resorption

Systemic-related resorption may be seen in patients with hyperparathyroidism.

Idiopathic Resorption

Occasionally teeth, typically first permanent molars, develop apical root resorption for which no cause can be elicited. These teeth have vital pulps and endodontic treatment does not arrest the condition and so is contraindicated.

MANAGEMENT OF CARIOUS TEETH

Pulp Protection

If a tooth is carious it is necessary to remove the carious dentine to prevent infection of the pulp. However this should be done in the way most likely to preserve pulp vitality. By removing the caries in several stages, it is often possible to preserve the vitality of a tooth, which, if the caries were excavated in one session, would have had its pulp exposed. The peripheral carious dentine and the central mass of caries are removed and a well-sealed interim dressing is applied. This process may be repeated as many times as necessary. Secondary dentine is expected to be laid down progressively as the caries is removed and dressings are applied. This treatment may take place over several months.

Partial Pulpotomy

If there is a small carious exposure in a permanent tooth it may be possible to perform a partial pulpotomy. After the removal of all softened carious dentine, a small cavity is cut at the exposure site with a diamond bur in a turbine to a depth of about 1.5 mm. The area is washed with sterile saline and haemorrhage is controlled, before a calcium hydroxide dressing or MTA is applied. The cavity is sealed with a reinforced zinc oxide–eugenol cement to ensure a good coronal seal.

ENDODONTIC TREATMENT OF MOLAR TEETH IN CHILDREN

With the increasing use of nonextraction orthodontic techniques and a lack of willingness of patients to lose their teeth, the demand for molar endodontics in young people is increasing. However, before root canal treatment is decided on, it is important to consider the whole dentition. For example, it would be unwise in a patient with unerupted or partially erupted second permanent molars to undertake root canal treatment of the first permanent molars. It is also most important to consider the long-term restorability of the tooth.

Endodontic treatment can present particular problems, not only because of the immaturity of the patient but also because of the immaturity of the tooth. Erupting lower molars are lingually tilted, making access more difficult. This can be disorientating when attempting to locate the canal orifices, especially the mesiobuccal orifice. Reactionary dentine is laid down from the coronal to the apical part of the root and is formed more rapidly in children, often making canal identification and coronal preparation more difficult. The apices may not be fully formed; in this situation the apex locator can be less accurate, and it is more difficult to control the length of the root filling. The dentine is softer than in adults facilitating procedural errors.

TEETH OF ABNORMAL FORM

Invaginated Teeth

Apical periodontitis may occur in two ways. The pulp space may become infected via the invagination, or the infection may spread from the invagination directly to the periradicular tissues without affecting the root canal. In the former case the tooth does not respond to sensitivity testing and root canal treatment should be undertaken in a modification of the normal method. In the latter case it may be possible to undertake 'root canal' treatment of the invagination without damaging the pulp (Fig. 11.16). Complex invaginations should be referred to a specialist.

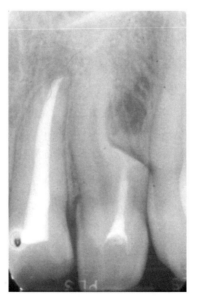

Figure 11.16

This invaginated maxillary lateral incisor tooth has been treated by 'root filling' the invagination. The pulp of the tooth is vital. From Pitt Ford HE (1998). Peri-radicular inflammation related to dens invaginatus treated without damaging the dental pulp. A case report. *International Journal of Paediatric Dentistry* **8:** 283–286, with permission.

Evaginated Teeth

Evaginated teeth tend to occur in the premolar teeth of people of mongoloid descent. There is a small outgrowth of tooth tissue from the crown (Fig. 11.17). This outgrowth usually contains pulp and tends to be fractured off during chewing, allowing infection to enter the pulp. The treatment of choice is to remove the evagination electively and perform a partial pulpotomy.

Talon Cusp

A talon cusp is similar to an evagination, but it usually affects incisor teeth (Fig. 11.18). The cusp may or may not contain pulp. Cusps may be unsightly or may interfere with the occlusion. They may be treated if required in a similar manner to an evaginated tooth. Any exposed dentine should be covered with restorative material.

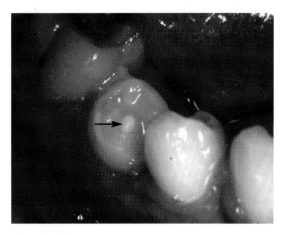

Figure 11.17

Evagination (arrow) affecting a mandibular second premolar.

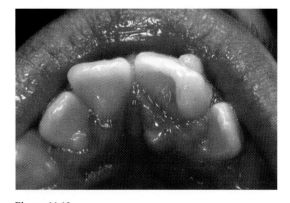

Figure 11.18

Talon cusps labially and palatally on a maxillary central incisor.

FURTHER READING

Dajani AS, Taubert KA, Wilson W, *et al.* (1997). Prevention of bacterial endocarditis. Recommendations by the American Heart Association. *Journal of the American Medical Association* **227**: 1794–1801. Available on-line at http://www.americanheart.org/Scientific/statements/1997/079701.html

Andreasen JO, Andreasen FM, Bakland LK, Flores MT (1999). *Traumatic Dental Injuries: A Manual.* Munksgaard, Copenhagen.

Cvek M (1978). A clinical report on partial pulpotomy and capping with calcium hydroxide in permanent incisors with complicated crown fracture. *Journal of Endodontics* **4**: 232–237.

Cvek M (1994). Endodontic management of traumatized teeth. In: Andreasen JO, Andreasen FM, eds. *Textbook and Colour Atlas of Traumatic Injuries to the Teeth*, 3rd edition, Munksgaard, Copenhagen: 517–585.

Dental Practice Board for England and Wales (1999). *National Clinical Guidelines and Policy Documents.* Treatment of avulsed teeth in children. Treatment of traumatically intruded permanent incisor teeth in children. Management and root canal treatment of non-vital immature permanent incisor teeth. Dental Practice Board, Eastbourne.

Fuks AB, Chosack A, Klein H, Eidelman E (1987). Partial pulpotomy as a treatment alternative for exposed pulps in crown-fractured permanent incisors. *Endodontics and Dental Traumatology* **3**: 100–102.

Jacobsen I (1980). Criteria for diagnosis in traumatised permanent incisors. *Scandinavian Journal of Dental Research* **88**: 306–312.

Leksell E, Ridell K, Cvek M, Mejare I (1996). Pulp exposure after stepwise versus direct complete excavation of deep carious lesions in young posterior permanent teeth. *Endodontics and Dental Traumatology* **12**: 192–196.

Mejare I, Cvek M (1993). Partial pulpotomy in young permanent teeth with deep carious lesions. *Endodontics and Dental Traumatology* **9**: 238–242.

Metzger Z, Solomonov M, Mass E (2001). Calcium hydroxide retention in wide root canals with flaring apices. *Dental Traumatology* **17**: 86–92.

Pitt Ford TR, Shabahang S (2002). Management of incompletely formed roots. In: Walton R, Torabinejad M, eds. *Principles and Practice of Endodontics*, 3rd edition, WB Saunders, Philadelphia: 388–404.

Sheehy EC, Roberts GJ (1997). Use of calcium hydroxide for apical barrier formation and healing in non-vital immature permanent teeth: a review. *British Dental Journal* **183**: 241–246.

12 ENDODONTIC EMERGENCIES

CONTENTS • Introduction • Reversible Pulpitis • Irreversible Pulpitis • Problems with Anaesthesia • Acute Apical Periodontitis • Acute Apical Abscess • Hypochlorite Accident • Flare-up During Treatment

INTRODUCTION

The treatment of endodontic emergencies can be difficult in the general practice environment, especially when the patient is in pain and the clinician is short of time.

REVERSIBLE PULPITIS

Signs and Symptoms

This is characterized by pain of short duration produced by extremes of temperature and sometimes by sweet food. The pain is normally of dentinal origin. No widening of the periodontal ligament space should be expected on radiological examination.

Look for:

- Exposed and sensitive dentine
- Caries
- Leaking restorations
- Recently placed restorations
- Cracks.

Treatment

Treatment involves removing the source of dentinal irritation. Sensitive dentine may be treated with fluoride resin or desensitizing toothpaste. Dental caries and leaking restorations should be removed and replaced with a sedative dressing. Recently placed restorations may need time to settle down; it is wise to check that there are no premature occlusal contacts. Teeth with cracks should be investigated. In small cavities a light-cured composite restoration may be useful, to prevent flexure of the fracture line. In some cases it may be necessary to prepare the tooth for a cast cusp-coverage restoration and to place a temporary crown.

IRREVERSIBLE PULPITIS

Signs and Symptoms

Persistent symptoms following reversible pulpitis may be indicative of irreversible pulpitis. There is an increased duration and intensity of pain. Spontaneous aching, throbbing and lingering pain, especially with hot stimuli, lasting several minutes or hours are common findings. Cold stimuli sometimes ease the pain. The offending tooth may be difficult to locate, and special tests could be required to isolate it.

Radiologically there may be early signs of periodontal ligament widening.

Look for:

- Extensive or recurrent caries
- Teeth with large deep restorations, or cast restorations
- Evidence of cracks or fractures.

If identification of the tooth is difficult, isolate the individual teeth with rubber dam and immerse each tooth in hot water.

Treatment

Ideal

The ideal treatment for irreversible pulpitis is to carry out complete cleaning and shaping of the root canal system. Sodium hypochlorite is used as an irrigant, and the canals are dressed with calcium hydroxide. The patient should be advised that the tooth could still be painful when the anaesthetic wears off. It may therefore be appropriate to prescribe analgesics, such as paracetamol (acetaminophen) 500 mg six times daily or ibuprofen 200–400 mg six times daily for 24 hours. The analgesics should be started immediately, before the anaesthetic begins to wear off. Sometimes using a longer-acting anaesthetic such as Marcaine (bupivacaine hydrochloride) is useful.

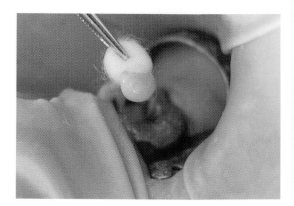

Figure 12.1

Sealing a corticosteroid dressing into the pulp chamber of a tooth with irreversible pulpitis. The root canals have not been instrumented.

When Time is Short

Remove all pulp tissue from the pulp chamber and irrigate with sodium hypochlorite. Do not instrument the canals. A corticosteroid preparation can be sealed in the pulp chamber with a temporary restoration of IRM (Intermediate Restorative Material: Dentsply, Weybridge, Surrey, UK: Fig. 12.1).

PROBLEMS WITH ANAESTHESIA

When attempting to root-treat a tooth that is pulpitic profound anaesthesia is important. Psychologically it is better for both the patient and the clinician to ensure good anaesthesia before embarking on treatment. It can be difficult to regain a patient's confidence if treatment has been painful. The patient can become more nervous, and will anticipate further pain with every slight vibration on the tooth.

The classic tooth that is difficult to anaesthetize is the mandibular molar; in this case the following regime may help:

* Give two inferior dental block injections
* A buccal and lingual infiltration
* Use intraligamental infiltration around the offending tooth (Fig. 12.2).

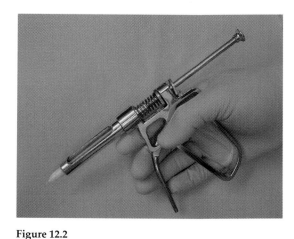

Figure 12.2

Intraligamental infiltration can be useful when anaesthesia is difficult to achieve.

If these still fail, intrapulpal anaesthesia can be useful. Use a slow-speed round bur to expose the pulp chamber. Warn the patient that the following injection will be painful for a just a few seconds. Insert the hypodermic needle into the pulp space and inject rapidly. Once anaesthesia has been achieved the pulp should be extirpated as efficiently as possible.

Maxillary molar teeth require both a buccal and a palatal infiltration in order to achieve adequate anaesthesia.

Intraosseous infiltration techniques can also be useful for pulpitic teeth, delivering local anaesthetic directly around the apices of the offending tooth.

Long-acting anaesthetics, such as marcaine, that last for 6–8 hours are useful in the treatment of very painful teeth. If the patient has been kept awake overnight with toothache then the longer duration of anaesthesia will allow him or her some respite.

ACUTE APICAL PERIODONTITIS

Signs and Symptoms

The tooth will often be painful to bite on and there will be tenderness over the apex of the tooth in the buccal sulcus. Radiologically there is usually widening of the periodontal ligament space.

Look for:

- Tenderness in the buccal sulcus
- Pain on palpation
- A darkened tooth, particularly at the neck
- Teeth with deep restorations or crowns
- A tooth that does not respond to pulp testing.

Treatment

Root canal treatment is required. The root canals must be completely cleaned, shaped and dressed. The tooth may need to be stabilized whilst cutting the access cavity, as the vibration when cutting can be uncomfortable. Sodium hypochlorite is used as an irrigant, and calcium hydroxide as the medicament after complete cleaning. The occlusion is adjusted to relieve any discomfort on biting.

Antibiotics are ineffective for the treatment of acute apical periodontitis if root canal treatment is not carried out. Therefore the practice of prescribing antibiotics instead of undertaking root canal treatment is not recommended, as pain will be prolonged. Analgesics may be required, and a combination of paracetamol (500 mg six times daily) and ibuprofen (200 mg six times daily) should be sufficient.

ACUTE APICAL ABSCESS

Signs and Symptoms

The abscess may develop from apical periodontitis or an exacerbation of a chronic periapical abscess. The tooth is exquisitely painful to touch, and may be extruded from its socket. There may be buccal swelling, which can be diffuse or fluctuant.

Treatment

To relieve the pain, drainage must be established, ideally through the root canal (Fig. 12.3). Following this full root canal treatment is carried out and the tooth is dressed with calcium hydroxide. Fluctuant buccal swellings may be incised to drain pus (Figs. 12.4–12.6). Teeth are generally not left open to drain unless there is an uncontrollable exudate, and then only for no more than 24 hours. Antibiotics may be required for a patient with systemic effects and a raised

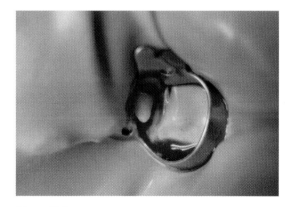

Figure 12.3

Drainage through the root canal of a tooth with an acute apical abscess.

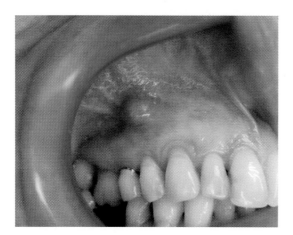

Figure 12.4

A fluctuant buccal swelling. The root canal system of the maxillary first premolar has been thoroughly cleaned and dressed with calcium hydroxide. The swelling is to be incised.

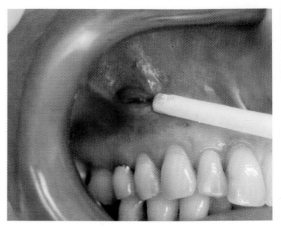

Figure 12.6

Pus has stopped discharging. Antibiotics would not be required in this case.

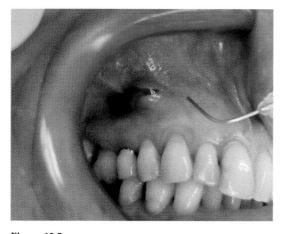

Figure 12.5

The swelling has been incised; a microsurgical aspiration tip is being used to remove pus.

temperature. Amoxycillin (250 mg three times daily) or metronidazole (200 mg three times daily) for three days should be sufficient. Some authorities recommend a single dose of 3 g amoxycillin. Analgesics may also be required. It is advisable to review all patients within 24 hours.

HYPOCHLORITE ACCIDENT

Signs and Symptoms

The patient will complain of severe pain while the root canal is being irrigated.

Look for:

- Immediate swelling
- Pain.

Treatment

A hypochlorite accident will greatly undermine the patient's confidence, and therefore the main emphasis must be on prevention. Always use an endodontic irrigating syringe (Fig. 12.7), measure the length of the needle (Fig. 12.8), inject slowly and do not allow the needle to bind.

If extrusion occurs:

- Stop irrigating immediately
- The best treatment is NO active intervention
- Extraction of the tooth is not indicated
- Use long-acting block anaesthesia to relieve the pain

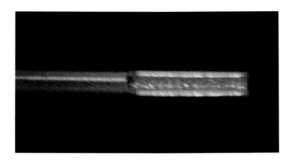

Figure 12.7

The tip of an endodontic irrigating syringe.

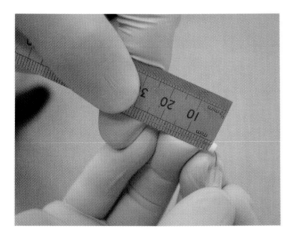

Figure 12.8

Measuring the irrigating needle to prevent extrusion of sodium hypochlorite.

- Prescribe paracetamol for pain relief
- Avoid aspirin (acetylsalicylic acid)
- Warn the patient that there is likely to be considerable swelling and bruising that is likely to last several days
- Follow up after 24 hours. In most cases there is total resolution; however in some affected tissues there may be abnormal feeling for some time.

FLARE-UP DURING TREATMENT

Common causes of flare-ups following root canal preparation are over-instrumentation, extrusion of irrigants or medicaments and leaving the tooth in a traumatic occlusion. With good technique these can be avoided.

Signs and Symptoms

The patient will usually complain of a continuous dull ache, and the tooth will be tender to touch.

Treatment

- Re-irrigate the canals with sodium hypochlorite
- Replace medicament and temporary restoration
- Check the occlusion. It may be necessary to remove the tooth completely from occlusion
- Analgesics may be required: 200–400 mg Ibuprofen six times daily.

Late flare-up (after 24 hours) occurs most commonly following instrumentation of teeth with pre-existing chronic lesions. It is as if the bacteria within the root canal system are 'stirred-up' by the cleaning process or perhaps inoculated through the apex. Perhaps a few viable bacteria remaining in fins or deltas are able to recolonize the root canal system. There is an exacerbation of the chronic condition, leading to an acute apical abscess, and treatment follows that for an acute apical abscess, already described.

Discomfort between appointments is also encountered with leaking coronal restorations. This should be considered when a tooth does not settle following thorough preparation, cleaning and medication. Microleakage will allow recontamination of the root canal system. Inadequate restorations should be removed prior to root canal treatment.

INDEX

Note: page references in *italics* refer to Figures; those in **bold** refer to Tables

abscess, apical, acute 24–5, *25*, 197–8
access cavity preparation 80–90
  aims 80
  depth estimation 81
  lid-off approach 80–90, *81*
  location 80
  preoperative radiograph 80, *80*
  troubleshooting 85–90
  unusual anatomy 87
acoustic microstreaming 139
AH 26 sealer 123
AH Plus sealer *123*
air abrasion 47, *48*
alveolar bone, anatomy 30
amalgam 159, *159*
  plugger 55, *55*, 85
amoxycillin 3
anaesthesia
  local 3, 14, 112
  problems with 196–7
  for procedures on maxillary teeth 168
  for procedures on mandibular teeth 168
Analytical Technology pulp tester 12, 13
anastomoses 27
angulation of the crown 87
ankylosis 7, *7*
antibiotics
  allergy to 1
  prophylaxis 3
anticurvature filing 97
apex locator 97–8, *98*
apical abscess, acute 24–5, *25*, 197–8
apical constriction *28*, 29
apical flare (stepback) 97, 103, 104
apical periodontitis 25, 79, 197
assessment 165–6
  patient's symptoms and signs 165
  radiological evidence of bony healing 165–6
  radiological review 166
asthma, as contraindication for surgical
      endodontics 166
avulsion 185–6, *186*

bacteraemia 3
bacteria 79, 112
balanced force action 96, 101–2, *101*

blockage 104–6
  prevention 104
  technique of managing 104–5
blood flow measurement 14
braiding 142, *143*, 144
Briault probe *12*, 85
bridge abutments 59–60
  sectioning 60, *60*
  removing 60
  root filled teeth 163
buccal sulcus, palpation of 8, *8*
burs 81, *83*, 87–8, 93, *93*, 95, 100, 101, 103, 134, 135

C-shaped canal 44
calcifications 85–6
calcium hydroxide 116, 117, *117*, 118, *118*, 121
  liners 50
  pastes 138
  points 119, *119*
  sealer 122
camphorated paramonochlorophenol 118
camphorated phenol 118
Cancellier 142, 143, *143*, 144
cancellous bone 30
cantilever bridge 151
carborundum disc 70, *70*
caries 46–7, *46*
  hardness 47, *47*
  management 48–51
    in non-vital tooth 51
    reason for 48–9
    technique 49–51
    teeth with destruction of marginal ridges 51
    timing 49
  paediatric 190–1
  recurrent 6, *6*, 7
  removal 47
cast cores 160
cast restoration 158
caulking 70
Cavi-endo endosonic insert *116*
Cavit 70
cavitation 139
cementum, anatomy 30
cermets 160
cervical resorption 175–7, *176*

chief complaint 3
children
    isolation for endodontic treatment 179–80
    management of carious teeth 190–1
    molar teeth 191
    root resorption 188–90
    teeth of abnormal form 191–2
    trauma 180–8
chisel, use in crown removal 58, *58*
chlorhexidine gluconate mouthwash 3, 112
chloropercha 124
circumferential filing 97
citric acid 113
clindamycin 3
cold lateral condensation 124, 125
cold testing 12, *13*
compomer 51
composite resin 50–1, *50*
    core 160, *160*
concussion 184
copalite varnish 49
copper bands 56
coronal flaring 139
coronal seal 45, *46*
cortical bone 30
cortical trephination 167
corticosteroid/antibiotic paste 117–18, *117*
cost post removal 145, *146*
cracked cusps, identifying 15–16
cracked teeth and fractures 51–3, *52–3*
crown-down preparation 100–2
    apical preparation 101
    coronal preparation 100–1
    rationale 100
    techniques 102–4
    use of Greater Taper files for 102
crown tapper 58, *59*
crowned teeth 56–9, *57–8*
crown fractures 181
    enamel or dentine fractures 181
    exposing the pulp 181–2
    lengthening 62, *62*
crowns
    metal-free 154–5
        anterior teeth requiring auxiliary retention
            155
        porcelain jacket crown 154–5
    with metal substructure 154
        metal ceramic crowns 154, 161, *161–2*
        metal composite crowns 154
    for posterior teeth 160–3
        cast metal 161
        ceramic 162
        full cast metal 161
        metal ceramic 161, *161–2*
        partial cast metal 161, *161*
        temporary 162

posts 155–8
    removing 57–9, *58–9*
    temporary 60–2
C-shaped canal 87, *87*
    in Mongoloid races 44
cuspal coverage restorations 158

debonding 152
dental tape 70
Dentatus screw posts 144, 160
Dentatus wrench 144, *145*
dentine, anatomy 27–8
    irritation 48
    peritubular 28
    primary 28
    secondary 28
dentine-bonding agents 50–1, *50*
dentine pins 78
DG16 probe *12*, 85, *85*
diabetes, as contraindication 1, 3, 166
diagnosis 23–5
diamond bur 70, 81, 87
drug abusers 3
Dry Dam 180
Dycal 181
dyes 87

EDTA (ethylene diaminetetraacetate) 86, 87, 104,
    112–13, *113*
Eggler post remover 146, *147*
elbows 96, *96*
electric pulp testing 12–13, *14*
endomethazone 138
Endoray 99, *99*
endosonic file 126–7, *127*
endosonic tip 128, *130*
endosonics
    gutta-percha removal using 140
    paste removing using 139
Endo-Z bur *84*, *85*
Enterococcus faecalis 79, 112
evaginated teeth 192, *192*
excavator 138
external resorption 188–90
extraction 137
Examination (extraoral) 4–5
Examination (intraoral) 5–12
    ease of access 5, *6*
    general condition of mouth 5–6
    mobility of fixed prosthodontics 8, *11*
    palpation of buccal sulcus 8, *8*
    percussion 7, *7*
    periodontal pocketing 8
    probing depth 8, *11*
    sinus tracts 8, *8*, *9*
    tenderness to palpation 7
    tooth mobility 6, *7*

facial swelling 4–5, *5*
File-eze *105*
filing 96–7
finger spreader 125, 126, 127–8, *127–8*
flare-ups during treatment 199
flat plastic in crown removal 58, *58*
Flexobend 103
Flexofiles 92, *92*, 102, 103
formaldehydes 118
fractured instrument 105, 141–4
    apical position 142–3, *143*
    coronal position 142, *142*
    immovable instruments 144
    middle position 143–4

Gates-Glidden burs 93, *93*, *95*, 100, 101, 103, 134, 135
    condensed gutta-percha removal using 140, *141*
    ledge formation using 104
    overuse 96, 106, *106*
    paste removal using 139
glass ionomer
    cement 51, 53, 55, *55*, 56, 150, 158, 160, 181
    sealer 123
Gonon post remover 146
Greater Taper files 102, *102*
Grossman's sealer 122
gutta percha 8, 10, 122, 124, 125, *125*, *126*
    condensed 140–1, *141*
    crinkling of 134, *135*
    custom-fitting a cone 126
    heat testing using 13, *13*
    removal 139–41, *141*
    removal of excess 128
    System B vertical compaction of 130–4, *131–3*

haemostasis 168
hand files 91–2
    instrument design 92
    ISO sizes and colours 91, **91**
    material 91
    placement of medicaments by 118–19, *118*
    restoring force 91–2
    taper 92
    tip design 91
    tip sizes 91
hand instruments 90–2
hand spreader 125, *125*
heart disease 3
heat testing 12, *13*
Hedstroem file 92, *92*, 96, 103, 139, 140, *141*
history taking 1–4
Howship's lacunae 30
hypertension, as contraindication for surgical endodontics 166
Hypocal 187
hypochlorite accident 198–9

ibuprofen 196
idiopathic resorption 190
immature tooth, trauma to 186–8
    filling the root canal 188
    treatment 186–7
    troubleshooting apical barrier induction 187–8
infective endocarditis
    as contraindication for surgical endodontics 166
    patients at risk of 3
    prevention 3
Intermediate Restorative Material (IRM) 147, 158, 168, 171, 181, 196
internal resorption 174–5, *174–5*
invaginated teeth 32, 191, *191*
iodine in potassium iodide 112, *113*, 117, *117*
irreversible pulpitis 24, 195–6
irrigants
    delivery 113–16
        endosonics 114–16, *115–16*
        syringe 113, *113–15*, 138
    types 111–13
irrigation, reason for 111
irritation dentine 48
isolation
    benefits 65
    reason for 65
    timing 65
    see also rubber dam

K3 rotary instruments *108*
Kalzinol 70
Ketac Endo sealer 123
Ketac Silver 160
K-file instruments 92
K-Flex files 92

Laser Doppler flowmetry 12, 14, *15*
lateral condensation 125–8
    cold 124, 125
    cone fitting 126, *126–7*
    custom-fitting a gutta percha cone 126
    removal of excess gutta percha 128
    see also warm lateral compaction
latex allergy 1, 65
length of canal
    estimation 97
    loss of 105
Leübke-Ochsenbein flap *169*
local anaesthetic 3, 14, 112
loupes 86, *86*
lubricants 70
Luxatemp 61, 152
luxation injuries 184–5
    extrusive 184
    intrusive 184
    lateral 184
lymph nodes, palpation of 4, *5*

lymphadenopathy of the submandibular lymph nodes 4

Machtou plugger 132–3, *133*, 188
mandibular canine, anatomy 40, *40*
mandibular first molar, anatomy 42–3, *42–3*
mandibular first premolar, anatomy 41, *41*
mandibular incisors, anatomy 38–40, *39–40*
mandibular second molar, anatomy 43–4, *43*
mandibular second premolar, anatomy 41–2, *41*
mandibular third molar, anatomy 44
Marcain 196
Masserann kit 144–5, *145*, *146*
master apical file (MAF) 103
maxillary canine 33, *33*
maxillary central incisor, anatomy 30–2, *32*
maxillary first molar, anatomy 36–8, *36–7*
maxillary first premolar, anatomy 33–5, *34*
maxillary lateral incisor, anatomy 32, *33*
maxillary second molar, anatomy 38, *39*
maxillary second premolar, anatomy 35–6, *35*
maxillary third molar, anatomy 38, *39*
medical history 1–2
medicaments 116–19
    intracanal 117–18
    placement 118–19
        calcium hydroxide points 119, *119*
        hand file 118–19, *118*
        spiral fillers 119, *119*
        syringe delivery 118, *118*
    reason for 116
    technique 117–19
mesio-occlusal cavities 158–9
mesio-occlusal-distal cavities 158–9
    cast restorations 159
    plastic restorations 159
metal shell crowns 56, *56*, 61
methacrylate resin 61
microcomputed tomography (MCT) *29*
microorganisms 79, 112
Mineral Trioxide Aggregate (MTA) 147, 168, 171, *172*, 182, 188
modified double-flare technique 103–4
    apical flaring (stepping back) 104
    coronal preparation 103
    preparation of the apical section 103–4

nasolabial folds, asymmetry 4, *5*
Nayyar core 150, 159, *159*
nerve fibres 27
nickel–titanium alloys 90, 92
    files 97
    orifice openers 93, *93*, 100
    rotary instruments 139
number of roots and canals 81, **82**

Obtura system 134, *134*, 150, 188

obturation 121–35
    criteria for 121
    root filling materials 123–4
    sealers 122–3
    techniques 124–34
        cold lateral condensation 124, 125
        System B vertical compaction of gutta percha 130–4, *131–3*
        thermocompaction (ultrasonic and mechanical) 124, *125*
        warm lateral condensation 124, *124*, 128–30, *129*
        warm vertical condensation 124, *124*
    troubleshooting 134–5
        crinkling of the gutta percha 134, *135*
        inability to place the spreader/plugger to length 135
        master cone will not fit to length 134–5
        removing cones during condensing 135
        voids in the obturating material 135
operating microscope 86, *86*
Oraseal putty 70, *71*
orifice shapers *95*, 96
orthodontic bands, placing 53–6, *54*
    reasons for 53–4
orthodontic extrusion 62–3
osteocytes 30
over-preparation 105

pain 24, 47
    from biting 16, *16*
    psychogenic 1
pain relief 168
palpation 4
    of buccal sulcus 8, *8*
    tenderness to 7
paracetamol 196
paraformaldehydes 118
partial pulpotomy 181–2, *181–2*
paste and cement root filling materials, removal 138–9
    removing paste from pulp chamber 138–9
    removing paste from root canals 139
    set cements 139
patency maintenance 97
percussion 7, *7*
perforation 96, *96*, 97, 104
periapical conditions 24–5, *25*
periapical inflammation, acute 24
periodontal ligament, anatomy 30, *30*
periodontal pocketing 8
periodontal probe *85*
periodontitis, apical 25, 79, 197
perio-endo lesions 173–4
phenols 118
Piezon unit *115*
plexus of Raschkow 27
pneumatic crown remover 58–9, *59*

poly acid-modified composite (compomer) 51
polycarbonate resin 47
post removal 144–7
    cost posts 145, *146*
    Masserann kit 144–5, *145*, *146*
    post removers 146, *147*
    screw posts 144
posts 88, 155–8
    cementing 158
    diameter 156
    direct cast post and core 157
    indirect cast post and cores 157
    length 155–6
    material 156
    post and core fabrication 157, *157*
    in posterior teeth 160
    preformed 157
    preparation of the post hole 157
    removal 144–7
    shape 155
    surface characteristics 156
preoperative mouthrinse 168
preparation, root canal
    access cavity preparation 80–90
    crown-down preparation 100–4
    hand 100–6
    instruments
        for apical preparation 107, *107–8*
        for coronal preparation 93, 107
        hand instruments 90–2
        rotary instruments 108–9
    mechanical preparation 106–9
        apical preparation 108
        avoidance of instrument fracture 107
        canal curvature 107
        coronal preparation 108
        cutting action 107
        merging middle section of canal 109
        pilot channel preparation 109
        rotation 106, *107*
    rationale 79–80
    techniques 93–9
        chemo-mechanical *94*
        crown-down preparation 93–6, *95*
        movement of files 96–100
        procedural errors 96
        terminology 93–6
pressure resorption 190
probing depth 8, *11*
Procera technique 155
Profile instruments *108*
prosthodontics, fixed, mobility of 8, *11*
Protemp 61, 152
pulp
    anatomy 27
    condition 23–4
    damage during preparation 47

necrosis 24, *24*, 47
    normal 23
    stones 85, *85*
    testing 12
pulp dentine complex 27
pulp floor map 85, 89
pulpitis 47, 53
    irreversible 24, 195–6
    reversible 24, 195
pyrexia 24

quarter-turn pull 97

radiographic film 17–18
    development 17–18, *18*
    film speed 17
    processing 17
    storage 17
radiography 16–23
    automatic processors 18
    digital radiography 18
    dose reduction 17
    fixing 18
    length estimation 98–9, *99*
    postoperative 171
    preoperative 80, *80*
    separating root canals 99
        mandibular incisors 99, *100*
        mandibular premolars 99
        mandibular molars 99, *100*
        maxillary premolars 99
        maxillary molars 99
    techniques 17, 18–23
        edentulous spaces 22
        retching 22, *23*
        shallow palate 22
        small mouth 22
    X-ray unit 16–17
Radix anchor post system 144, *156*
reamers 91–2
    instrument design 92
    ISO sizes and colours 91, **91**
    material 91
    restoring force 91–2
    taper 92
    tip design 91
    tip sizes 91
recapitulation 97
recementing a cast restoration or post crown 164
reciprocating action 97
replacement resorption 189–90, *190*
resin sealers 123
resorption
    cervical 175–7, *176*
    external 188–90
    internal 174–5, *174–5*
    pressure 190

resorption *continued*
  replacement 189–90, *190*
  surface 188
restorations 87–8
  anterior teeth 152
  cuspal coverage restorations 158
  extensive restoration 154
  internal bleaching 153, *153*
  mesio-occlusal cavities 158
  mesio-occlusal-distal cavities 158–9
  occlusal loading 151
  posterior teeth 158
  preservation of tooth substance 151, *151*
  restorability 151–2
  severely broken-down teeth 159–63
  simple restoration 153–4, *153*
  timing 152
  treatment planning 150–1
retreatment, root canal 137–48
  gutta-percha removal 139–41, *141*
  illumination and magnification 138, *138*
  ledges 147
  paste and cement root filling materials 138–9
  perforations 147–8, *148*
  post removal 144–7
  preparation of root canals 148
  reason for 137–8
  silver points and fractured instruments 141–4
  single cone gutta-percha removal 139–40
  technique 138
  Thermafil 141
  timing 138
reversible pulpitis 24, 195
rheumatic fever 3
Rinn holder paralleling device *19, 20–1, 23*
root canals
  anatomy 28–30, *28*
  location of extra 88–90
    four canals in mandibular molars 89–90, *89*
    second mesiobuccal of maxillary molars 88–9, *88–9*
    two canals in a mandibular premolar 90, *90*
    two canals in mandibular incisors 90, *90*
root end surgery 137
root filling materials 123–4
root fracture
  horizontal 182–4
  longitudinal *16*, 51–3, *52*, 166, *166*
root resorption *see* resorption
rubber dam
  badly broken-down teeth 77–8, *77*
  bridges 77, *78*
  clamps 66–8, **69**, 78, 179
  forceps 68–70, *70*
  frames 66, *66–7*
  isolation problems 77–8
  kit 71, *72*

multiple teeth isolation 75, *75*
placement 71, *71–2*, 75
punch 68, *68–9*
quick single tooth isolation method 73–4, *73–4*
sealants 70–1, 179
sheet *71–2*
silicone 65, *66*
split-dam technique 76
using wingless clamps 76–7, *77*
varieties 65, *66*
Wedgets, use of 70, *70*, 180
Ruddle post remover 146, *147*

Schick system (digital radiography) *19*
Schilder plugger 132–3
sclerosed canals 86–7
Sealapex 123
sealers 122–3
sealing access cavity 149–50
sectioning, crown removal and 59, *59*
severely broken-down teeth 159–63
silver point removal 141–4
  apical position 142–3, *143*
  coronal position 142, *142*
  middle position 143–4
sinus tract 5, *6*, 8, *8*, *9*
sodium hypochlorite 80, 98, 111–12, *112*, 148
Spencer Wells forceps 99
spiral fillers 119, *119*
stepback (apical flare) 97, 103, 104
stepdown technique of canal preparation 103
  apical flare (stepback) 103
  initial coronal flare 103
  precurving files 103
Stieglitz forceps 140, *140*
strip perforation 96, *96*
Stropko irrigator 85, *85, 86*
subluxation 184
Super EBA (ethoxybenzoic acid) 147, 168, 171
surface resorption 188
surgical endodontics 166–73
  anaesthesia, pain control and haemostasis 168
  apical surgery 167
    apical curettage 167
    root-end surgery 167
  corrective surgery 167
    perforation repair 167
    root resection 167
    tooth resection 167
  flap design and reflection 168–9
  flap replacement 172, *172*
  incision and drainage 167
  indications 166–7
  osseous entry 169–70, *169–70*
  postoperative instructions 172–3
  postoperative radiograph 171
  root-end filling 171, *171–2*

root-end resection and cavity preparation 170–1,
 171
surgical armamentarium 167–8
surgical sieve 1
System B vertical compaction of gutta percha
 130–4, *131–3*
 backfill 134, *134*
 cone fit 132
 down pack 134
 fitting the cone 133
 measuring the plugger 132–3, *133*
systemic-related resorption 190

talon cusp 192, *192*
teeth of abnormal form 191–2
Tenax titanium post kit *155*
test cavity, cutting 15
Thermafil 141
thermal tests 12
thermocompaction (ultrasonic and mechanical)
 124, *125*
tooth mobility 6, *7*
Tooth Slooth 16, *16*, 55
transient apical breakdown 185
transillumination with fibre optic light *15*
transportation 96, *96*, 104
trauma 180–8
 diagnosis 180–1

troubleshooting
 apical barrier induction 187–8
 obturation 134–5
 root canal preparation 104–6
 blockage 104–6
 fractured instrument 105
 loss of length 105
 over-preparation 105
 perforation 104
 transportation 104
 wine-bottle effect 106
Tubliseal 122
tubular sclerosis 48
tungsten carbide bur 81, 87

ultrasonic tip 87, 90, 138, *139*, 144, *144*, *171*
ultrasonics in crown removal 58, *58*

varnish 49

warm lateral condensation 124, *124*, 128–30, *129*
warm vertical condensation 124, *124*

zinc oxide and eugenol
 cement 50, *50*, 53, 61, 70, 138, 147, *150*, 158, 181, 186
 sealers 122
zinc phosphate cement *54*, 56, 78
zips 96, *96*, 97